SET FREE & SATISFIED

"A fresh, humorous, positive approach for those struggling with eating issues. Grab some friends and study this book together. In moving from isolation to community you will discover healing and a new freedom."

—Susan Alexander Yates, speaker and author of *Risky Faith: Becoming Brave Enough to Trust the God Who Is Bigger than Your World*

"Joy offers a compassionate, practical, and Christ-centered approach to finding freedom from disordered eating. She candidly and winsomely shares about her own journey towards freedom, inviting readers along with her through her tried-and-true Releasity program. She gives encouragement to depend on the Holy Spirit for true freedom that lasts. It's a book I'm grateful for personally and professionally."

—Heather D. Nelson, Christian counselor and author of *Unashamed: Healing our Brokenness and Finding Freedom from Shame*

"*Set Free & Satisfied* is brilliant. Joy tackles a complicated problem with humor and honest experience. She guides the readers with refreshing, God-centered grace. I can see this program helping many people who currently feel alone in their struggles with overeating. I can't wait to share it with my patients."

—Faison Green Knox, MD

"Our relationship with food goes deeper than our mouths and appetites. I appreciate how Joy, with her wit and candor, invites you to come and connect with her through personal stories, Scripture, cognitive behavioral therapy, and real-life practical tips to address the struggle of overeating. *Set Free & Satisfied* compels and equips the participant to take time and really sit with what is going on in their heart, mind, and soul. Joy's and previous participants' stories encourage the reader to realize that change can occur, food struggles are released, and lasting healing and freedom in Jesus Christ are found. Jump in with a friend, surrender, give yourself time and space to really reflect on what Joy is offering for you. You will be glad that you took the journey!"

—Jennifer Harris, MS, Registered Dietitian-Nutritionist

"AHHHH ... *Set Free & Satisfied* is a welcome and necessary perspective for nourishing our bodies in these hurried times. Joy masterfully shares well-earned wisdom on how to weave healthy eating habits into our lives. Rooted in Scripture, her voice soothes and reflects the kind whispers of our Creator and ultimate healer, God our Father. Whether you are challenged with weight issues or not, her story will move you to a deeper belief that God always has a creative plan to bring light to our struggles."

—Catherine Farley, PT, MPT, Wellness & Writing Coach, author of *Desert to Dawn, Reflections to Inspire, Refresh & Renew*

"*Set Free & Satisfied* is filled with HOPE for the weary dieter and for those who long to stop overeating. The practical step-by-step approach is set apart from others by the powerful Scripture truths shared throughout. As a health professional, this book is invaluable to me in counseling both individuals and groups in breaking free from the cycle of food restriction and overeating."

—Heather Sylvester, MA,
Registered Dietitian-Nutritionist

"Mast has written a powerful guide to help those struggling with food addiction in a relatable way with clear actionable steps. Her Christian worldview points to the powerful One who designed us and His intricate and deliberate design of the human body. In doing so, she provides an excellent way to connect or reconnect with our inborn hunger and fullness signals. This book provides clear guidance and support to help individuals on their journey to freedom."

—Beth Butler, MD

"*Set Free & Satisfied* is a faith-based book that takes you on a journey of finding freedom from overeating. Joy Mast provides clear teaching and practical steps, while also sharing her own struggles and healing journey. With a voice of understanding, she helps the reader feel supported and not alone in this journey. We've had great success offering the Releasity course to women in a group setting at our church, too!"

—Catherine Nations, Women's Ministry Director,
Carmel Baptist Church, Matthews, NC

"With its perfect balance of gospel-centered grace and practical guidance, *Set Free & Satisfied* is a must-read for anyone who loves Jesus and struggles with overeating. Its pages contain a treasure trove of emotionally healthy wisdom and resources, thoughtfully laid out to guide you step-by-step into the process of long-term heart and life change. Joy humbly and humorously shares bits and pieces of her own journey in a way that makes her readers feel both understood and inspired. For the discouraged readers who have tried numerous methods for overcoming their struggle with food, *Set Free & Satisfied* reminds us that we serve the God of Hope (Romans 15:13)."

—Bethany McGuire, MA, Christian Counselor

"*Set Free & Satisfied* takes us on a journey of hope, healing, and transformation in our relationship with food. Joy shares her painful struggle with emotional eating in an authentic, relatable, and honest way while showing us how spiritual, mental, and emotional healing will lead to freedom from overeating. She provides us with a step-by-step plan to align our thoughts, actions, and habits with a healthy mindset. This book provides valuable tools and insights that will inspire change from the inside out, leading to a peace-filled approach to food for long-term health and well-being."

—Sarah Duncan, RN NBC-HWC,
National Board Certified Health
and Wellness Coach

"Joy offers us a better posture to benefit from the Lord's healing, a healing that is more lasting than any weight loss program. She reminds us that God has created masterpieces in us all and to start in the middle, in the heart, will be where the true healing begins. Joy reminds us that our God is a healer and wants to offer us all a lasting freedom. She turns our attention towards a God who has the capacity to help us see things differently – from brokenness to healing to newness of life. By returning to the biblical text, these pages point us to an ancient model of healing."

—John Rogers, MDiv, Director, Peterson House

"Rooted in Christ's love for us, Joy Starnes Mast offers a hopeful path into freedom from our unhealthy relationship with food. Her vulnerability, sound Scripture references, and practical guides are among the reasons why I recommend *Set Free & Satisfied*."

—Stephen E. Davis, MDiv, Anglican Priest (ACNA)

"This relatable book, filled with personal stories from the author, leaves me with hope for the now and the future, as well as with helpful tools as I move forward in my journey with emotions and food. After almost a lifetime of diets and gimmicks, I am relieved at age sixty-two to find a new path that offers freedom with healthy boundaries that I am eager to explore. All that I have read in this book gives me what I need to move from isolation and poor choices and has opened my eyes, mind, and heart to ways of living abundantly that I have never before considered."

—Kathy Fletcher, Releasity participant

"Joy Mast has beautifully created a strategic guide for helping others pursue freedom from the stronghold of emotional eating. I only wish her book had been available to me twenty-five years ago! In my years of searching for help relating to my health and wellbeing, I haven't encountered a book as relatable and practical as this one. It is a resource that I will return to as well as recommend to others."

—Eliza Johnson, Releasity participant

Set Free & Satisfied

A RELEASITY  RESOURCE

Set Free & Satisfied

A Grace-Filled Guide to Stop Overeating
and Start Fully Living

JOY STARNES MAST

SET FREE & SATISFIED

Copyright © 2023 by Joy Starnes Mast

www.joymast.com

All rights reserved. No part of this book may be reproduced, stored in a retrieval system, or transmitted in any form or by any means without the prior written permission of the author.

For information email: joy@joymast.com

The advice contained within this book does not constitute or serve as a substitute for professional medical or psychological treatment, therapy, or other types of professional advice or intervention.

Scriptures taken from the Holy Bible, New International Version®, NIV®. Copyright © 1973, 1978, 1984, 2011 by Biblica, Inc.™ Used by permission of Zondervan. All rights reserved worldwide. www.zondervan.com. The "NIV" and "New International Version" are trademarks registered in the United States Patent and Trademark Office by Biblica, Inc.™

Published in the United States by Somersby Press

Cover design by Steven Mast

Interior design by Kim Hall

ISBN: 979-8-9878883-0-8

Dedicated in loving memory to my father,
Clarence Starnes Jr.,
the first person to show me compassion
in my struggle with overeating.
Tucking me in one night, he sat at the edge of my bed
and told me he knew how I felt.
In that moment, I felt loved, seen, and not alone.

For you, the reader, I hope this book shows you how
your heavenly Father also loves you, sees you and is
with you. May the words on these pages build
communities of connection and a greater bond between
you and your Maker.

CONTENTS

CHAPTER 1
My Story and Your Story 3

CHAPTER 2
Remember What You Want 23

CHAPTER 3
Expect the Lord to Heal 41

CHAPTER 4
Live Out of Your Freedom 67

CHAPTER 5
Eat with Hunger When You Feel It 89

CHAPTER 6
Acknowledge Your Emotions 113

CHAPTER 7
Seek the Spirit Every Day 133

CHAPTER 8
Experience Life to the Full 155

Next Steps 185
Additional Resources 188
Acknowledgments 197

INTRODUCTION

After years of wrestling with compulsive overeating, God set me free. Through many channels like counseling sessions, support groups, meeting with friends who shared my journey, prayer, and Scripture, God brought healing that has resulted in a long-term transformation in my life and in my relationship with food. While weight loss has resulted from this healing, more importantly, God has used the experience to bring me closer to Him.

During the healing process, I discovered concepts that were completely foreign to me—namely, that I had freedom to eat any kind of food, that I have an internal hunger/fullness cueing system to guide my eating, that I was going to food for comfort rather than effectively coping with my emotions, and finally, that God wasn't mad at me for all these missteps. He simply wanted me to come to Him instead of running to excess food. In those dark days, I began considering the fact that surely other women out there were as misguided as me when it came to health and disordered eating. I vowed to help those women if I ever found my way out.

Thankfully, God healed me. In 2012, I wrote the first Releasity course, inviting women to my home to explore these concepts in a group setting. Since then, the course has been offered in churches and online. More than once, women enthusiastically shared the material with friends in another city or state. That encouraged me to convert this course to a book, so women anywhere can find freedom from their own pattern of overeating.

In his *New York Times* bestseller, *Atomic Habits,* author James Clear states the importance of establishing systems for meeting our goals, rather than solely focusing on the goal itself. He argues that both teams in a game want the highest score at the end, but neither team will win by simply staring at the score on the scoreboard. Instead, the steps they've taken to prepare and play the game are more likely to help them win.[1] Releasity also follows a system or sequence of steps (outlined below) that encapsulate my discoveries along the healing path.

My hope is that you'll grab a friend (or a few) and dig into this book to discover the truths of God's freedom-giving approach to eating. Life has too many wonderful avenues to explore for us to be stuck in our misery of overeating and feeling regret over our choices. May you release this problem to God and find yourself released!

THE BUILDING BLOCKS OF RELEASITY

In the nine-week Releasity course, we use two important acronyms as a guide.

RELEASE: Seven Ongoing Steps to Freedom

Remember What You Want.
Expect the Lord to Heal.
Live Out of Your Freedom.
Eat with Hunger When You Feel It.
Acknowledge Your Emotions.
Seek the Spirit Every Day.
Experience Life to the Full.

The last four steps are easily recalled using the acronym **HELP**:

Hunger—Wait for **hunger** before eating.
Emotions—Name your **emotions** when you want to eat but aren't hungry.
Lord—Take your emotions to the **Lord** in prayer.
Pursue life—Find other activities to **pursue** while you wait for physical hunger to return.

CHAPTER 1

My Story and Your Story

I have called you friends, for everything that I learned from my Father I have made known to you.
—John 15:15b

This book starts with an ending—my father's funeral. Like me, he was very social, and a large crowd gathered to pay their respects on the night of his funeral visitation. People stood in line for hours in a line that wound through every room of that large funeral home and spilled out onto the sidewalk in the historic district of my hometown.

I'm told that my friends from college and high school ended up in the line together and, in their small talk, someone looked up a set of stairs and pondered aloud, "I wonder what's up there?"

When my comedic friend April replied, "Heaven," they all broke out in laughter. I like to think my dad was laughing with them, too, because I sure hope you get to witness your friends and family gather to celebrate you after you die. What started as a two-hour visitation window stretched beyond four hours, and we were there much longer than planned.

Amid the sea of people who came through and shook the hands of my family members, telling us what my dad had meant to them, a local pastor friend appeared. Bruce had a great sense of humor, and I was glad to reconnect with him.

"Joy," he said, "I've got some good news and some bad news."

"What's that?" I said, a little surprised at his comment because most people just started by telling me how sorry they were for my loss.

"The good news is that a lot of people loved your dad. The bad news is they're all here tonight!"

We immediately started laughing together in a way that marked appreciation for my dad and provided some much-needed levity. It brings tears to my eyes even now as I write it.

In your struggle with food, you might feel like I did that night. It's hard, it's been going on a while, and you'd be happy to wrap it up any time soon. You vacillate between wanting to give up and wanting to keep going with managing your weight because you know it's important. In fact, an article from the Boston Medical Center claimed that an estimated forty-five million Americans go on a diet each year, yet two-thirds of Americans are overweight or obese.[1] We live in the tension of these two worlds: trying yet failing. For some reason, you haven't given up 100 percent, and for some reason, you have enough hope to start reading this book. So like my friend Bruce, I have some good news and some bad news for you.

The good news is that you're probably going to read something in this book that you haven't tried before. Something is going to spark a change in how you eat and think about food, and it will likely impact you for the rest of your life.

Now for the bad news: this change won't happen overnight.

The concepts in this book—steps to finding freedom from over-eating—are a culmination of what God has shown me about my own problem with overeating. Initially, I thought I simply needed to make some superficial, behavioral changes to bring my eating under control. But God showed me that it's an inside-out job. Lasting change happens when God starts the change in our hearts by address-ing the underlying conditions that lead us to overeat in the first place.

When it comes to my history with food, I'm comparable to Serena Williams or Tiger Woods—a super-athlete who began her training at a young age. While others were training in some useful skill, I was growing in my overeating and in my size! I escaped to food when I felt bored or lonely and continued this habit into adulthood. However, I didn't realize those were the things that led me to overeat. I just knew I was always overweight enough to garner criticism from peers and loved ones.

In high school, I met a girl named Amy who would drive me to aerobics, and she'd talk openly about the problem of how much she loved food. She'd make it funny, and we'd laugh. For the first time, I began enjoying the freedom of friendship with someone who shared my struggle. I began learning the power of community to address this area, and it's one of the reasons I value the community aspect of the Releasity course when it takes place in person.

Along with Amy, I've had other friends throughout the years who have exercised with me. Their company helped me to show up for myself and move my body in beneficial ways. If you're dealing with overeating, I wish this for you, too—a friend you can talk and walk with. You may have picked up this book in isolation, but I hope you'll contact someone you trust and read it with them.

By my early twenties, I'd had some on and off success with dieting, usually prompted by the pending deadline of a friend's wedding and an unflattering bridesmaid's dress I'd be forced to wear in front of a crowd. I'd take off some weight, then put it back on. Apparently, I wasn't alone. Research shared by the Cleveland Clinic noted that 80 to 95 percent of dieters regain their weight.[2] Like the popular joke, I'd keep losing weight, but it would keep finding me. Over time, I developed a bit of insanity around dieting and eventually restricted myself to the point of developing some even more disturbing eating behavior. I'd secretly sneak food and, around the age of twenty-five, I knew I needed help.

It was 2001, and I'd spent the past two years sharing a three-story house with two other women while working as a speech pathologist at the Children's Hospital in Washington, DC. My housemates and I had our friendships with one another and enjoyed loose connections with each other's friends. One night, I came home from work and discovered a line of cars parked along the street in front of our house. *Oh, that's right*, I thought. *Margaret's friends are coming over to hang out after work tonight.* Even though I liked her friends, their gathering didn't involve me, and I planned on grabbing my dinner and making myself scarce. This was a typical weeknight in the life of a young professional.

I greeted Margaret's friends, then made my way to the kitchen to prepare a quick dinner before heading up to my room. Her friends had gathered in the den adjacent to the dining room, so I set my dinner plate on the table and planned to eat quickly as they talked. With the women at my back, I looked around the table for something to occupy my mind and eyes as I ate my green beans. I put a bite in my mouth and noticed a large, important-looking book entitled *The Harvard Guide to Women's Health* sitting on the table. I figured that a woman in the group must have brought it by to show someone else. Lucky for me, I had it all to myself for the time being. I'd do a little research on my new food-sneaking problem.

This habit mostly occurred in the secret back portion of my kitchen and in my dark car at night. I had figured out that if I snuck into our tiny galley pantry behind the kitchen, I could easily keep an eye on the food I was surveying as well as the doorway to the kitchen in case someone came in and found me. I always looked for something sweet and had even started anticipating these moments and planning for them at the end of a long day. It took me back to being a kid when I'd scour our cabinets for something tasty. My mom worked at the local hospital just to put food on the table in the first place, so I spent afternoons alone at home and figured out ways to eat sweets, even if we didn't have cookies in the house. I poured extra sugar on my cereal, for example, and poured chocolate chips on a spoonful of peanut butter. I even recreated a recipe I found in a 4-H cookbook by stacking a marshmallow on a peanut butter cracker and putting them in the newly invented microwave for ten seconds to warm the marshmallow. Back then, I did such things because I was bored and liked sugary treats, but I didn't know that yet.

Now, however, I was an adult. Why was I still secretly eating so much? Why did it not stop in my pantry? Why did I drive to the local Giant supermarket and buy myself an entire box of Oreos, plus a half-gallon of milk, then secretly consume them? I was getting concerned. Why was I eating all these sweets when I didn't want to be eating them? At least, that's what I told myself—I didn't want to be eating them. That was the problem. I kept shoving food in my mouth, despite my mind telling me to stop. I'd begun to wonder if I had some type of official eating disorder. I knew it wasn't anorexia because I liked eating too much to severely limit my caloric intake. I knew it wasn't bulimia because I was too chicken to make myself bring up the excess food I had consumed.

This Harvard medical guide offered me the chance to grab a quick diagnosis (this was before the days when you could turn to Google or WebMD). If anyone stepped in the room and saw what I was doing, I was prepared to avoid embarrassment and quickly turn the page to any topic other than eating—skin growths, incontinence, whatever! My shameful habit had kept me in isolation so far, and I wasn't ready to change that.

I found the chapter that covered eating disorders and quickly searched for my ailment. My eyes followed the topic through headings and paragraphs. *Anorexia Nervosa*—no. *Bulimic Nervosa*—no. *Binge Eating Disorder* . . . maybe? Who knew this was even a thing? The official medical definition of binge eating was the "consumption of large quantities of food in a short period of time." Bingo. The book recommended I seek professional help.

I closed the book, headed to my bedroom, and decided to contact the only counseling office I knew of in the DC area. The psychiatrist who started the clinic had recently taught a class at my church and had encouraged us to not hide behind our false selves. I've always valued authenticity, so his message resonated with me. He'd also taught at fancy universities like Harvard, Yale, and Georgetown. Unfortunately, I did still care about superficial things like my image. If I was going to be treated for an eating problem, I figured it would be best to hire a therapist as dignified and distinguished as possible.

After hearing my concerns, the intake coordinator paired me with a woman named Patti. I arrived at her office one day after work and heard water flowing in the waiting room as I took my seat. Later, I came to realize that most counseling offices have these tabletop water fountains that give off a soothing sound for anxious people like me. Either that, or they at least muffle the true confessions people are sharing behind closed doors. I filled out the new-patient paperwork, pausing when I reached a question I'd never seen before in a medical office.

What is your view of God?

No theologically sophisticated answer came to me. I sighed as my eyes teared up and I wrote, "I love Him. I just love Him."

In fact, I was hoping God and Patti could get me out of this pit, since I was beginning to believe I couldn't do it alone.

Another thought hit me as I waited for my first session with Patti: *That's it. I'm officially screwed up*. All I'd wanted was to lose some weight over the years, to avoid spoken or unspoken criticism of my body by fitting into medium-sized clothing, whether it be a skirt for a night out on the town or a swimsuit when I convened with college friends for our annual lake trip. But after spending my youth overeating and overweight, now I was at risk of—or perhaps had already developed—a bona fide eating disorder. I'd seen results with some diets, but they never lasted. No short-term weight loss stuck, nor did it undo years of sadness linked to others' hurtful comments and the embarrassment of having my oversized body on display in front of others. No matter my success, I would always remember my otherwise very loving grandmother standing over my sixth-grade, awkward self as she debated with her best friend whether or not my "fat" was just "baby fat."

"When is she going to lose the fat?" she asked her friend.

"It's baby fat," her friend replied, trying to comfort her (no one expressed interest in comforting me, mind you).

"No, it's not baby fat! She's in sixth grade!" my grandmother lamented.

It's also hard to forget the time a sales associate coached my mom in what types of swimsuits she should buy me to hide the unflattering, pudgier parts of my body. "You see that piece of fat there? That's what you want to cover up," she said as she pointed to the piece of flesh that bulged at the front of my armpits.

Losing weight or gaining weight, not having sweets or having too many, the hole I had dug over the years was deep, and I had now landed in a shrink's office to try and handle it.

I spent the next several months meeting with Patti. She began to uncover some of my false beliefs around which foods were okay to eat and which foods weren't, how I gave food and my body size too much power over my life, and how I'd unconsciously made a habit of eating sweets to not feel sadness about the parts of my life I couldn't fix. I moved away from DC a year later and had to leave Patti behind (this was before the era of Zoom calls). That left my food issues and the deeper question of why I consumed excess food and how to break the cycle unresolved.

The night I looked for a diagnosis in the Harvard health guide, I had no idea how long it would take to fix my problem. I assumed that in the same way I sometimes counted calories, limited my eating, and lost some weight, the long-term solution would also be superficial. I certainly did not expect a deep excavation of "why" I overate in the first place. I didn't anticipate a years-long process of learning how to take my pain to God instead of the kitchen, nor could I imagine building an arsenal of fun, life-giving activities to explore as alternatives to exploring my pantry to soothe my pain.

My full transformation came through meeting with more counselors, joining support groups, reading books by various authors, meeting with friends who shared my experience, meditating on Scripture, and spending time in intentional prayer over multiple years. It included nights when I cried myself to sleep and mornings when I watched my tears drip into my coffee cup just moments after the coffee had dripped into the pot. There were more bingeing episodes, though they didn't happen as often as the years passed. Eventually, thank God, the bingeing stopped. Thankfully, so did my feelings of shame and self-loathing.

In the process, I discovered healing concepts in the Bible that were completely unknown to me when I began my search for help with binge eating. If I hadn't known these truths, surely other Christians didn't know them either, I reasoned. Inspired by women like Harriet Tubman, who helped others find freedom after she achieved her own, I felt a strong compulsion on my path to food freedom. I vowed that if I ever found my way out, I would help other women find their way out as well.

Five years after the binge eating and self-destructive thought patterns stopped, my father died. Our family gathered around his hospital bed in his last minutes of life, staring down the machines that would let us know when his heart had finally stopped beating. As his minister prayed and gathered us close like a hen with her chicks, I became painfully aware of my dad's passing and that each person's life has an end date. If I really wanted to help people who struggled with food issues like I had (and like many of my family members before me), I had to begin the work. Possibly in an attempt to avoid my own grieving, I began writing a course called "Releasity" and invited six friends to come to my house to take it. The key concepts that helped me heal would become the focus of our biweekly sessions.

Since then, the Releasity class has been held in churches and online. It is a unique space where women can be with each other and

Jesus and talk about overeating. Honestly, I always considered the process as one in which God releases us from our problem (hence the name), but a recent participant named Laura changed my thinking. The point of it all, she said, is for us to "release this" to God. From there, He releases us.

The steps of that process are highlighted in the acronym RELEASE, which will be the basis of each chapter in this book. After the first three steps of RELEASE, we will also move into practical steps that can be easily remembered on a daily basis through the acronym HELP, which stands for "hunger, emotions, Lord, and pursue life." As we ask God to help us, these four aspects set the stage for our daily rhythm of following God and being healed.

Women have told me that I talk too fast in the course and that they don't have enough time to write down everything I'm saying. For a while, I wondered why they felt like they had to catch everything, until it hit me. This is a fresh perspective, and the hope it gives is energizing! Some women would call a sister or friend in another city or state and share the content with them. Across the miles, they partnered to find freedom using the biblical concepts of the Releasity course. As I grew more convinced of the merit behind this God-centered approach, I realized it might be worth putting the content into a book so it could be used anywhere, whether or not I was present. In the same way the Harvard health book started me in the right direction, I hope this book will help you begin to approach your eating in a new way. After you've finished reading it, I encourage you to read books by authors with similar approaches to eating. Beyond that, I'm thrilled to give credit to God through this teaching that shows the wonders He can work.

If you've had your fill of not only food but also shame, guilt, regret, and isolation, this book is for you. I assure you God has an escape plan for you. It's not a superficial solution and it won't be the "fast fix" I hoped for when I first peeked in that health book, but trust me, it's the solution you want. Authentic and long-lasting, this approach will bring you closer to the God who loves you. He isn't mad at you; rather, He longs to help you.

Are you ready to move on with your life and stop constantly thinking about what you look like, what you weigh, and what you're eating? I know I was. I believe this book will hold a fresh perspective for you because it's not your typical diet book. In fact, it's not a diet book at all! Diets, with their rules and restrictions, can dangerously backfire. Diets are what led me to see a counselor in the first place. They're also the reason I firmly believe in an eating mindset that starts with our God-given freedom. This new approach to eating is gentle and judgment-free. Releasity's many mental, emotional, and spiritual benefits will positively impact your whole life, not just how you eat or what you look like.

If you'd like some evidence of how this book is unique, the following is a list of outcomes reported by Releasity course participants over the years. See if any of the feedback sounds like where you currently are or where you'd like to be.

- Instead of feeling hopeless, you can feel hopeful that God can make you new.

- Instead of always fighting the desire to overeat, your desire can change to wanting to eat in a way that is beneficial for you. You can even follow through on those new desires with ease, eventually.

- Instead of feeling shame and beating yourself up for your eating habits, you'll learn how to be curious, not critical toward yourself. With gentle awareness, you'll become a kind cheerleader for yourself.

- Instead of external food rules and diets controlling you and making you miserable, you can discover the freedom God has for you while you follow your internal hunger and fullness cues.

- Instead of isolating yourself because of this food issue, you'll learn to share about your struggles in a safe relationship where you feel supported and heard.

- Instead of obsessively thinking about food, your body, your eating habits, or your weight, your mind can be transformed to have biblical, noble, and worthwhile thoughts!

- Instead of ineffectively using food to cope with your problems and uncomfortable emotions, you'll learn how to effectively cope with life's pain points.

- Instead of depending on yourself for change, you'll learn to lean on the Holy Spirit's power to transform you and set you free from overeating.

- Instead of feeling far from God because of the distance this food problem has caused, you can return to God's "throne of grace with confidence" (Hebrews 4:16) and have greater intimacy with the Lord than you've had before.

- Instead of wasting hours, days, weeks, and months thinking about your body, you'll learn new and enjoyable ways to spend your time and get your mind off of food.

WHAT ABOUT THE WEIGHT?

You may have noticed that losing weight is not mentioned in the list above. In reality, women who eat excessively don't necessarily need to lose weight. Overeating and the preoccupation with food and body isn't reserved for those who carry extra pounds on their frame. However, if you are in a position where you would medically benefit from carrying less weight, the Releasity approach can also help you. I have lost and kept off over forty pounds since discovering the principles contained in these pages. Better yet, I know I have freedom to eat any kind of food I want and don't beat myself up when I occasionally make a food choice that isn't beneficial for my body.

God has more for you to experience and enjoy in life, and I'm convinced that He does not want us to be obsessed with how much we eat, how much we weigh, or what we look like. When we as women learn to follow our internal hunger/fullness cues, cope with our emotions in ways that don't involve food, and find other joyful ways to spend our time when we aren't physically hungry, our bodies eventually reach an "ideal weight" for our genetically determined frame. The Releasity approach can show you how to address the underlying cause of your overeating and clear a path for you to go to God for solutions to your actual problems. As you go to food for its proper function, your weight will find its rightful place.

BETTER TOGETHER

The comfort and insight I gained from other people on my healing journey cannot be overstated. I couldn't have found my path to freedom without the company, conversation, and support of others who knew how I felt. If you've picked up this book with a plan to read it alone, I implore you to find a friend or two to read it with you. Each chapter ends with reflection questions to stir your conversations.

Be patient, and be hopeful. You are making a fresh start on your journey to healing.

MY STORY AND YOUR STORY

REFLECTION QUESTIONS

After reading each chapter, take time to process the chapter and answer these questions on your own. Later, share your answers as part of a group discussion or with a friend who is also reading the book.

Jot down the key ideas covered in this chapter.

_____

_____

_____

_____

If your struggle with food has been going on for a while, what are some ways that you have previously tried to manage your eating without success?

_____

_____

_____

_____

Why is managing your health important to you? List some reasons.

_____

_____

_____

_____

Who are some friends or loved ones with whom you feel safe sharing this area of concern? Name a friend or two who might be willing to pray for you in this area.

_____

_____

_____

_____

In terms of your eating habits, what are some ways that, before now, you have experienced shame or have been too embarrassed to share with others?

_____

_____

_____

_____

JOURNALING

At the end of each chapter in this book, you'll have the opportunity to set a timer and write your thoughts for a few minutes. Before you move ahead, take a moment to write any new insights, thoughts, or reflections you had after reading this chapter.

_____

_____

_____

_____

_____

_____

MEMORIZE

Each chapter will contain a verse for you to memorize and meditate on. It's helpful to use a spiral index-card ring to keep your verses in one place. Begin by writing the following verse about God's guidance on an index card:

"I will instruct you and teach you in the way you should go; I will counsel you with my loving eye on you."
—Psalm 32:8

PRAYER

Each chapter will hold a space for you to pray at the end of your reading. As we begin, let me pray for you.

Dear God, I pray that each person reading this book will find healing and freedom as they seek your guidance in this area of their lives. Give them the courage to be honest, the patience to take every step needed, and the strength and companionship they need to persevere. Thank you that you are with them and you see them.

Amen.

PRACTICE

Finally, you'll have the opportunity to put each chapter's concept into practice at the conclusion of each chapter. For now, keep to the path you're on. Continue reading!

CHAPTER 2

Remember What You Want

Where there is no vision, the people perish.
—Proverbs 29:18

Years ago, I traveled to the North Carolina mountains with my extended family. The women divided up responsibilities for meal prep, and since I was thirty-two weeks pregnant, everyone felt sorry for me and assigned me one simple task: preparing a dessert for the Saturday evening meal. I'm not sure why I didn't make the dessert in advance—that was my first mistake. Second, and worse, I forgot a key ingredient and didn't realize it until I started baking the dessert. I had to dash into town from our cabin to grab baking soda from the local grocer.

Walking into the small, dimly lit store, I felt like I'd stepped back in time forty years. I couldn't find what I needed, so I searched for an employee. I found a manager helping another customer purchase cigarettes. He was unlocking a glass cabinet that contained carton upon carton of cigarettes. As I waited my turn, I couldn't help but hear their conversation. The manager handed the customer his preferred cigarette brand and the shopper about fell over in shock.

"Man!" he shouted in disgust. "The price of these cigarettes is killin' me!"

I had to laugh. Wasn't the man more at risk of dying from the tobacco than from the price of the cigarettes? Current studies indicate that over sixteen million Americans have a smoking-related illness,[1] so I think my assumption was right. If I had a smoking habit, I know I'd be more far concerned about death than the dollar sign on the cigarettes.

As I waddled out of the store and carefully inserted my pregnant body back into the car, I gave more thought to this shopper's comment and realized something. We all have our own perceptions of our problems. When it comes to food, what might be a problem for you may not be the same problem someone else faces with overeating. You might just want to lose some weight so your clothes aren't as tight. Another person may want to lose weight so they can go on trips and walk long sightseeing distances with their friends and family or go upstairs without panting breathlessly by the time they reach the top. Whatever negative habit we've acquired, be it smoking or overeating, we are entitled to have different perceptions of how our problem uniquely affects us.

Since you've picked up a book about overeating, let me ask you: What is killing you when it comes to overeating? Is it the cost of the food? Is it the impact it's having on your health? Is it because you lack energy for your daily tasks? Could it be that you don't have the money to replace an entire wardrobe of clothes that don't fit? It helps to reflect on the problems that overeating have caused in your life. As you embark on a new way of living and eating, identify what you "want" instead of focusing on "the problem."

This is Step One of Releasity: **Remember What You Want**. In moments of temptation, if we can remember what we really desire—be it better health, freedom from fixating on our bodies, or comfortable clothes—instead of excess food, we may be able to resist the temptation.

Recognizing the problem helps us turn our "problems" into positive "I want" statements that can provide us with a positive vision for the future. For example, if you struggle with being out of breath when you walk, remember that you want to be able to walk easily without huffing and puffing. Identifying your desire gives you a vision for your future that will help you persevere. This helps you stay focused on why you want the change, so you can pray about it and stay aware of your habits as you go about your day. I can't tell you how many times I thought I cared about my eating issues but, in truth, I completely forgot about the new way I wanted to live on a regular basis. A simple Post-it Note with my reasons for wanting to make the change would have been helpful.

Recognizing the problems we face in order to remember what we want has a few benefits. First, it removes distraction and reminds us that we care about this area of our lives. We are then able to focus on our true desire instead of the problem we have named. Furthermore, it helps keep our eyes off (and our noses out of) other people's business. This is important, because it's not uncommon for overeaters to overly concern themselves with the flaws or needs of others instead of focusing on the change needed in their own lives. I spent years trying to help fix others while denying my own need for growth. Looking inward rather than outward helps us identify our unique pain points in this area to stay motivated.

Second, shifting our focus to the core problem helps us get back on track after a setback. Those setbacks are normal, but they don't have to ruin us! Instead of beating ourselves up for not fitting into our clothes, the experience of realizing our jeans are too tight can become an opportunity for a helpful reminder. Instead of saying, "I'm so sick of my jeans not fitting!" we say, "Oh, that's right, I wanted to make changes with my eating so that my jeans can fit." We feel thankful that we are "recognizing the problem" and remembering the new life we desire. Instead of feeling badly about ourselves, we experience a positive moment of remembering why we care. That becomes a catalyst for us to pursue change and persevere.

LOCUSTS? YEP, LOCUSTS

It's important to stay hopeful as you explore the challenges you've faced due to overeating. Many of us are discouraged after years of trying and failing to lose weight. To maintain a positive mindset, let's start with one of God's promises.

In the Bible, we read about the Israelites, a group of people who lived in a place called Judah about six hundred years before Jesus lived on the earth. At one point, the Israelites had a serious problem with locusts. In case you're not familiar with locusts, let me assure you that the sight of them is downright disturbing. If spiders give you the creeps, then trust me, you don't want anything to do with locusts. Shaped like grasshoppers, they can be as long as six inches and will suddenly attack an entire area by swarming.

A prophet named Joel tried to comfort the Israelites by telling them God would take care of them after a swarm of locusts had caused significant damage in their lives. Joel 2:25–26 reflects God's words to the Israelites: "I will repay you for the years the locusts have eaten—the great locust and the young locust, the other locusts and the locust swarm—my great army that I sent among you. You will have plenty to eat, until you are full, and you will praise the name of the Lord your God, who has worked wonders for you; never again will my people be shamed."

Did you notice the list of locusts? The passage includes great ones, young ones, and even a locust swarm. The problems in our lives related to overeating are similar to all those locusts—they come in many forms. Thankfully, God promised that He would come and make up for the years the locusts had eaten. God said He would work wonders and remove the shame of these people who suffered from locust damage. Does this make you think of the harm that's occurred in your own life as a result of eating too much?

If so, how would you assess the damage? In case you're tempted to think that your biggest problem is the number on the scale (that is, if you even weigh yourself), let me suggest that the scale doesn't tell the whole story. Solely focusing on "the number" means we neglect to explore all the areas of our lives that can be improved if we start to follow God's guidance for our eating and our lifestyle habits. In fact, our issues with food have implications that don't relate to how much we weigh. The excess food we eat can affect our way of living, elicit hurtful comments from family members, and drain our energy.

DAMAGE OTHERS CAN SEE

Let's start with the locust damage *others can see*. Carrying extra weight causes pain and physical discomfort in our bodies. I've heard women talk about difficulty breathing, lack of energy, and pain in their knees, legs, and feet that they believe is related to overeating. As a child, I developed a painful rash between my upper legs because my thighs rubbed together when I walked. In college, I figured out that rubbing deodorant between my thighs helped prevent the chafing. This was a brilliant solution!

Another type of locust damage is how overeating can limit our activities. As a kid in gym class, I never understood why they called one of our required runs the "300-yard dash." I certainly wasn't "dashing" anywhere! I was always a slow runner and the last to finish. My embarrassment might have been alleviated if the class had moved on without me to their next exercise. But no. They often gathered in a group and waited out my last moments of misery, watching me slowly pull up the rear for our class. In particular, I remember the day my best friend and teacher continued to cheer for me long after my friend had finished. I'd made the mistake of wearing a Myrtle Beach T-shirt that day, and my friend and the teacher kept shouting, "Come on, Myrtle! You can do it!" I knew they were comparing me to an elderly lady who couldn't run fast, and I hated every minute of it.

My most frightening and visible locust damage came on a ski slope shortly after I finished college. I'd signed up for a trip with friends even though I was out of shape and overweight. I had no idea how to ski but, being the hopeless extrovert that I am, I joined the group anyway and hoped for the best. Bad idea. Our lodge was located across the road from a ski lift, but my friends assured me I could just ride the lift down to my beginner ski class. Getting on the ski lift was no problem—you just sit down, and I am really good at sitting. The trouble started when we neared the exit landing. My friend Vanessa said, "Okay, Joy, just hold your skis out in front of you and glide onto the snow as we come up to the top."

Before I knew it, I was lying on the ground at the edge of the lift with three of my friends standing over me. They shouted instructions on how to lift myself up, but I had no coordination and no upper body strength to get the job done. I honestly can't remember how I got into a standing position, but I do remember looking down the mountain and thinking there was no way I would make it to the bottom alive.

God bless Vanessa, who at one time had been a kids' ski instructor. She offered to help me, and to this day, I feel overwhelming gratitude for her kindness and her Wonder Woman ability to usher me down the mountain with my arms around her waist and my skis tucked parallel inside her skis. With four poles in her hands and two hundred extra pounds of me leaning on her back, she accomplished a miraculous feat in delivering me to my first ski class.

Maybe your story isn't as dramatic as my ski-slope disaster, but has overeating prevented you from enjoying physical activities? Women taking the Releasity course have shared a variety of problems related to "visible damage." For example, their clothes are too tight or don't fit anymore (which creates a financial strain when they have to replace them). They feel self-conscious about how they look in the clothes that do fit and tend to add more layers to hide their body, which leaves them feeling uncomfortably hot. They hate shopping.

The physical toll of overeating includes increased weight gain, arthritis, shortness of breath, the inability to walk far or uphill without pain, high blood pressure, and elevated cholesterol levels. Women find it a problem that weight-related medical issues force them to go on medication. They have fears for their future health. One woman shared that she becomes sweaty with little exertion and that it's hard to get up and down from the floor when playing with her grandchildren. Some women regret that they can't be as active as they once were and that exercise is now hard for them. Others share how overeating depletes them of energy and leaves them exhausted, limiting their motivation to prepare meals. Their budget stretches thin due to eating out because they don't cook meals at home.

Another type of visible locust damage is how our overeating affects our relationships. One Releasity participant shared that her husband is disappointed with her and wants her to be thinner and healthier. He believes this will help them live a longer life together. We might also receive unwanted comments about what our bodies look like. Those wounds stick with us. One such memory for me is from junior high summer camp. It was the day of "team building" and our group had to balance on a large log that hung from a tree. As the group brainstormed ways to accomplish this, one boy shouted out, "Let's start by putting the heaviest people in the middle. Joy, get on!" We all knew he was right, and I obediently took his orders to help our group achieve its goal.

DAMAGE OTHERS CANNOT SEE

Beyond the problems that others can see is a world of invisible problems. First of all, a range of emotions accompanies overeating. We feel shame and embarrassment after people's negative comments or simply from our own perceptions of ourselves. We feel insecure about how we look and experience self-hatred, guilt, and negative thoughts about ourselves. We are hard on ourselves and very short on grace and mercy, which is exactly what we need. Women taking the

Releasity course have shared feelings of isolation, as well as weariness and loss of hope after many failed attempts with weight loss. On top of the emotional roller coaster, women have shared about the guilt they felt for adding insult to injury when they "ate their emotions" instead of feeling them.

A young mom of three discussed how overeating caused her to feel irritable toward her family members. This is true for many of us, because when we're frustrated with our eating habits or the number on the scale, we can be bad-tempered for the rest of the day. Often, our family members take the brunt of this frustration because we lack patience with them when we can't attain what we want with our bodies.

Our eating habits can make us feel afraid. We may be concerned about future medical issues or ones already diagnosed. We fear trying new things or doing group activities where our weight will be put on display or limit our ability to participate. I remember a time in my life when, if I was invited to do something active, my first thought was, *Will anyone else going be as out of shape as I am?* I didn't want to be the only one struggling to keep up. If you have children, you know the fear of passing your tendency to overeat to your children. *If I sneak food, will they?*

Speaking of sneaking, how about the behaviors that are exhausting to hide? We binge in secret. We buy food from the grocery store that we have to conceal from others, so we furtively eat it between the store and home. After the binge, we deprive ourselves of food for a while hoping to undo the damage. This pattern of bingeing and restricting becomes a covert life.

Mental preoccupation with food is another type of locust damage. Some days I became so obsessed with my weight that I would step on the scale multiple times between breakfast and bedtime. I also kept a daily count of the calories I had consumed on a dry-erase board in my kitchen. When we are mentally consumed like this, even "success" isn't satisfying. I once lost a significant amount of weight (albeit temporarily) and went to a Gap store to buy a new pair of shorts. Approaching the counter to pay for my size-six shorts, I simply couldn't believe the number on the tag was accurate. With a suspicious tone, I asked the sales associate, "Is Gap sizing their shorts differently now?" She looked at me with a confused expression and said, "I don't think so." As I pressed the issue, I'm pretty sure she was thinking, *No, crazy lady, but please take your new size-six shorts and get out of here.* Mental bondage is miserable when you're obsessed with food and your body.

THE GREATEST LOCUST

The last locust is the greatest one of all. It's simply the fact that we have an overeating problem, and no matter how much we try, we cannot fix it, or at least we can't fix it for the long-term. We are stuck between wanting the food and not wanting it and never make any lasting progress. We love the moment of pleasure when we give in to the food we crave, but we hate how we feel and the consequences we experience afterward. We go from the pleasure of the food's taste to the embarrassment of a bloated face, all because we ate more sugar than we needed.

Throughout my disordered eating, I often felt defeated because I had no self-control. I assumed God wanted me to take care of the one body He gave me, but I was failing at that. Inside, another battle was raging. Depending on the moment, I often felt like I wanted food and/or thinness more than I wanted God in my life. As a Christian, that felt terrible to admit. How self-centered and self-serving could

I be? I was a walking contradiction, doing things I didn't want to be doing. The life I said I wanted to be living, I wasn't living at all. I simply couldn't make long-term weight loss happen, and I couldn't beat off all the other negative tendencies that came with overeating, like hating myself and obsessing over my body. I desperately wanted change, but I had no idea how to achieve it.

In the middle of this food struggle, and a few months after I said "goodbye" to my counselor Patti, I spent a summer training to be a missionary. During a teaching session, the leader read a Bible passage from the book of Romans, in which Paul, an early missionary of the church, wrote, "I do not understand what I do. For what I want to do I do not do, but what I hate I do" (Romans 7:15). The passage continues, "For I have the desire to do what is good, but I cannot carry it out. For I do not do the good I want to do, but the evil I do not want to do—this I keep on doing" (Romans 7:18–19).

When the teacher finished reading, he asked the group, "Who does this sound like?" (He probably thought one of us missionary trainees would recognize the author as Paul.) From my seat in the back of the room, I accidentally blurted out, "Me—it sounds like me!" My friends and I laughed out loud, which got the teacher's attention. He asked what had set off the laughter, and when everyone pointed at me, I told him what I'd said. Genuinely amused by my comment, he asked what had made me say it. Familiar with my food problem by now, I answered as effortlessly as I've ever articulated anything: "Because I wake up with good intentions, and I go to bed with regrets."

Does that sound like you? Do your good intentions deteriorate as the day wears on? If so, maybe you'll appreciate the end of Paul's words on the subject. Romans 7:24–25 says, "What a wretched man

I am! Who will rescue me from this body that is subject to death? Thanks be to God, who delivers me though Jesus Christ our Lord!"

That's it. Jesus Christ is the ticket to finding our way out of this overeating issue. The same God who told the Israelites he would **restore** to them the years the locusts had eaten will also **deliver** you from your dilemma of relying on food for comfort. If you're open to letting God heal you through this process, keep reading. If you're not a Christian, don't stop reading. Consider the possibility that a relationship with your Creator might be the key that finally helps you overcome your food issues. Stick with me and keep turning the pages. You might be pleasantly surprised.

No matter the damage others can see, the damage they can't see, or the fact that we can't fix ourselves, God wants us to be incredibly hopeful because He's in the business of restoring and delivering. If He was able to set me free from my food addiction, I'm confident He can move powerfully in your struggle with food and bring you lasting freedom. God will do a new thing in your life, just as he promised the Israelites in Isaiah 43:19 when He said, "See, I am doing a new thing! Now it springs up; do you not perceive it? I am making a way in the wilderness and streams in the wasteland."

You are investing the time to read this book, and God will honor the fact that you have come to Him for help. Recognizing the problems that have resulted from overeating and naming what we want in place of them is the first step toward healing.

REMEMBER WHAT YOU WANT

REFLECTION QUESTIONS

Jot down the key ideas covered in this chapter.

_____

_____

_____

_____

What were your thoughts in response to the story about the man who complained that the prices of the cigarettes were killing him?

_____

_____

_____

_____

Three reasons were given for "recognizing the problem": remembering that we care about this overeating problem and that we want change, focusing on our own problems (rather than trying to fix other people), and having a positive starting place when we make mistakes with food. Which of these reasons seem particularly beneficial for you? What are some other reasons it's helpful to "recognize the problem" with overeating?

_____

_____

_____

_____

SET FREE & SATISFIED

A variety of problems related to overeating were named, including physical ailments, others' hurtful comments, negative internal emotions, and obsessive thoughts about our eating and weight. What problems did you identify with as you read this chapter?

_____

_____

_____

_____

This chapter highlights the grandest locust of all, which we are incapable of fixing ourselves, despite knowing so much about our eating problem. Even though we want change, we also want the moment's pleasure of indulging in more food than we are hungry for. What are some inconsistencies you have seen in your own life when it comes to having certain behaviors with food that contradict what you think or feel?

_____

_____

_____

_____

JOURNALING

Set a timer for five minutes and write some of the problems in your life that have resulted from your overeating. What are your locusts? Think about the visible and invisible ones.

Use the chart below to write your "Locust List," then make a corresponding "What I Want" list to name the things you hope will happen as you begin to eat differently and become healthier. These might relate to your physical health, your external appearance, how you want to feel about food and/or yourself, things you want to do, or relationships you want to work on.

List of Locusts	"I want _____" Statements
Example: It hurts my knees to go upstairs.	Example: I want to be able to go upstairs without pain.

MEMORIZE

After each chapter, take some time to choose a verse (or use the verse provided below) and memorize it during the week. Write the verse on a Post-it Note and display it where you can see it regularly, or keep a spiral index-card ring where you can gather the verses in one place.

"Forget the former things; do not dwell on the past. See, I am doing a new thing! Now it springs up; do you not perceive it? I am making a way in the wilderness and streams in the wasteland."
—Isaiah 43:18

Copy this verse in the space below as you begin to commit it to memory. If you choose a different verse, write it in the space below.

_____

_____

_____

_____

_____

PRAYER

Think about whether there might be a friend who shares your experience who could walk this journey with you. Maybe she could read along with you and you could pray for each other specifically in the area of healing from overeating. Perhaps there is someone you trust to be encouraging in this area who will also pray for you. Ask them to regularly pray for your healing around overeating. For now, write your own prayer to God in the space below.

_____

_____

_____

_____

_____

_____

_____

PRACTICE

It's important to begin showing yourself love and self-care. While it may feel overwhelming to completely overhaul the way you eat and exercise, take time this week to care for your body in smaller, practical ways. In doing so, you are communicating to yourself that your body is worthy of being cared for. Drink a tall glass of water first thing in the morning, floss your teeth, or moisturize your body using a lotion you like.

CHAPTER 3

Expect the Lord to Heal

Lord my God, I called to you for help, and you healed me.
—Psalm 30:2

I grew up on a farm in North Carolina and when I left for college, I kept the thick drawl I acquired being raised in a rural Southern community. My new college friends had great fun listening to the unusual ways I pronounced words—when they weren't busy trying to figure out what I'd actually said in the first place. Freshman year, I met a guy named Michael Beal, but I pronounced it Michael "Bill" because of my thick accent. This went on for a good number of months, if not a whole year, until my friend Anna saw his name in writing somewhere.

"Joy," she said. "His name is Michael *Bee-uhl*, not Michael Bill!"

"I know," I said. "Michael Bill."

"Joy, look at how it's written. B-E-A-L is pronounced *Bee-uhl*, not *Bill*."

I kept agreeing with her, not realizing that my pronunciation of "Bill" was any different from hers. As she continued to teach me kindergarten-level phonetics, it dawned on me how I'd made the mistake. In my recollection, my kindergarten teacher had taught us that the words "mill" and "meal" were rhyming homonyms, pronounced the exact same but with different meanings. I'm blaming it on the teacher, though she may have a different viewpoint on this.

Did you believe something as a child that turned out not to be true? Apart from Santa, the Easter Bunny, and the Tooth Fairy, what have you falsely believed in? For example, I used to think that all men drove trucks and all women drove sedans because that's how it was in my rural community. For a long time, my friend Laurie was convinced that there was always an ocean behind a long row of high-rise buildings, because that's what she experienced every time her family drove to the beach.

As we think about the next step of Releasity, **Expect the Lord to Heal**, let's consider misconceptions we've had about God. I used to believe He was like Santa—you be good, and He'll be good to you. If you're not good, you're going to have to explain to everybody those lumps of coal that have accumulated in your life because of your bad choices. Apparently, I came away from my childhood education with some false information, including the fact that I had to be good and moral for God to like me. What inaccurate beliefs have you had about God?

Many Christians would say they intellectually agree with what the Bible says about God, that He's always loving, helpful, and wanting to heal people. But I don't think we necessarily believe this when it comes to our food problem. This could be the case for various reasons. You may think your overeating problem isn't a big enough crisis for God. With the despair and legitimate emergencies in so many corners of the world, it's tempting to think, *Why would God care about my food issues?*

A Releasity participant named Anna shared her biggest breakthrough in the program was realizing that she didn't need to have a natural-disaster-level problem in order to ask God for help; she could come to Him asking for relief from her overeating. Others of us may feel distant from God, either because He hasn't delivered us from our food problem before and we're angry at Him, or because we think He's mad at us for how we've wrecked our bodies with our lack of self-control. We might think it's vain to bring our weight and health issues to God or that He doesn't care about them. We could even think the issue has a "statute of limitations," like the warranty on a dishwasher, and at this point we've let the problem go on too long for God to fix it. You likely have additional or different reasons why you think God might not want to help you.

Do you ever feel like that with God? Do you ever think He's upset with you over your food problem? On a scale of 1 to 5, how much do you really believe God 1) *can* and 2) *will* heal you of your overeating? Choosing 5 means you fully expect Him to heal you and 1 means you don't believe He can or will. Pause to answer this question. The results are telling and can help you process your perception of God. Do you believe God can heal you and will heal you?

I have observed in several women a lack of belief that God will bring positive change in their lives in the area of food, if it even occurs to them to consider bringing it to God in the first place. We must address the barriers to believing God will help us if we are to confidently move forward in this process. In Releasity, we EXPECT that He will help us because this approach to food is not self-help; it's Holy Spirit help.

ENCOUNTERING GOD

In my healing journey with food, I began by asking God to help me lose weight, simply because somehow, He gave me the grace to believe He would. My first encounter with the real, living God was at a Bible study in college. I hadn't planned on doing anything Bible-related in college. My mom had mentioned InterVarsity Christian Fellowship while she was writing the check for my dorm room. I remember thinking, *Poor Mom, she doesn't know what people really do in college.* I planned to party and put faith on the back burner.

However, when I arrived in Chapel Hill the fall of my freshman year, InterVarsity was hosting a free pizza party for the girls in my dorm. Free pizza was all I needed to change my mind and join the Christians at their gathering. It turned out their plan was to feed us, then invite us back to Bible study. Not wanting to be rude, I visited the first study and felt overwhelmed by God's love in a way that caused me to begin sobbing in front of this entire group of people I didn't even know. I would later realize this experience was a Holy Spirit encounter, but at the time, it was enough to keep me engaged in InterVarsity. From there, I slowly began to explore a relationship with this loving, personal God.

The summer after college graduation, my friend Anna got engaged and asked me to be a bridesmaid. She knew I was insecure about my weight, so she made a point to take me on a walk and break the news to me that her bridesmaids' dresses would be sleeveless. As we walked the gravel path in Winston-Salem where I'd stopped to visit her on my way to graduate school, she said, "I know you don't wear sleeveless shirts because you're self-conscious about your arms, so I'm giving you a year to mentally and physically prepare for it."

I did what any desperate and decently God-fearing person does. I bought a journal and began writing my prayers asking for help. Each one always started with, "Dear God, please help me lose weight." I had no time to waste on any other polite or flowery intro. God did help me lose some weight before Anna's wedding, but years later, when my restrictive dieting had led to uncontrollable binge eating, I realized on a deeper level that I believed He'd grown weary of helping me in this area. I feared my problem would outlast his kindness. I was creeping toward His help's expiration date, convinced that the longer I screwed up, the less He would be willing to intervene.

But that's not who God is. God had to show me His everlasting, never-expiring love and willingness to help me. I had to align my thoughts with His thoughts because they aren't the same. Tim Keller, the late pastor of Redeemer Church in New York, said it well: "It is easy to fall into the trap of thinking that God's love and concern for us rise and fall according to how well we are doing in living the Christian life. After all, we ourselves frequently give and withdraw our love from others depending on whether they are living in a way that is pleasing to us. Thankfully, even though we are marked by inconsistency, God is marked by constancy."[1]

As you **Expect the Lord to Heal**, try to answer three important questions:

1. Why can I expect God to heal me?

2. How will God heal me?

3. What is my responsibility in all this?

I once accepted a position as a youth minister, and let's just say I was ill-qualified to assume this leadership role. I'd never been a youth minister, and though wonderful people helped me, it was a stressful job and I wasn't good at it for a very long time. At our first group meeting, a young and overly confident student raised his hand in front of everyone and informed me, "You're going to have to make this a whole lot more fun if you want people to come back!" I wanted to say, "Good idea. Next week, let's play pin the tail on . . . what's your name again?"

My perfectionism and focus on all my failures, plus my loneliness and hopelessness from still being single at age thirty, sent me into a clinical form of anxiety and depression. Many days, on my way to work, I'd walk by a dilapidated home that reminded me of an old haunted house. The unpainted shutters hung crooked, and the grass in the yard was perpetually neglected. I often thought the house resembled how I felt during those years—run-down and forsaken.

Two years later, when my youth ministry job had become much more rewarding and my depression had subsided owing to prayer, counseling, and medication, I received an invitation to the home of one of my students. I was shocked to discover that the address he gave me led to the same "spooky" house I'd passed so many times. During those two years, the family had been renovating the home from the inside out, and when I entered the house, I could see the beautiful work they had already completed. From the inside out, that old home was becoming a masterpiece, but you wouldn't know it from an exterior view. I always appreciated that house because it showed me how God transforms us—the change He brings in our lives always starts from the inside with our hearts.

In the same way that house needed a renovation, we need restoration when it comes to our relationship with food. God knows this.

And if we need it, God will do it! Jesus said in Matthew 6:8, "Your Father knows what you need before you ask him." Likewise, Paul wrote to the Philippians, "My God will meet all your needs according to the riches of his glory in Christ Jesus" (Philippians 4:19).

God knows we need intimacy with Him to live a life of flourishing. Jesus said, "If you remain in me and I in you, you will bear much fruit; apart from me you can do nothing" (John 15:5). God will heal us from overeating because it will lead us to intimacy with Him. Hebrews 12:2 says of Jesus, "For the joy set before him, he endured the cross, scorning its shame, and sat down at the right hand of the throne of God." Many agree that "the joy set before Jesus" was the connection we would have with God because Jesus's death removed the sin that separates us from a perfect God. Jesus died for us because God wants to be with us forever! However, when we go to food for comfort and companionship rather than going to God, we prevent ourselves from connecting with God in the way He intended. Why wouldn't He help us break this unhealthy cycle of trusting food for connection and comfort, if it means we can have more connection and intimacy with Him?

Another reason God will heal us is so we can live in freedom. Isaiah 61:1 prophesied that Jesus would come "to proclaim freedom for the captives," and that means freedom from all sorts of bondage. For those of us who overeat, there's a lot of setting free God can do! He can set us free from the actual overeating. He can set us free from obsessive thoughts about what we are eating now or what we will eat in three hours. He can set us free from believing our bodies are flawed and from the constant waves of criticism toward our bodies. He can even set us free from the pain we've felt when others have verbally criticized our bodies. Some of these hurts may have been inflicted by someone who isn't even alive anymore. The pain of past wounds that once led us to overeat can become a powerless memory as God gives us freedom.

God-given liberation from overeating also opens the way for us to have powerful connections with people, rather than being tied to something as lifeless, and as temporarily satisfying, as food. When we stop turning to excess food for comfort and companionship, we find the time and energy to pursue healthy bonds with people and enjoy a variety of enriching activities and experiences. We are set free to pursue life beyond food. Our world and our communities offer so many interests, outlets, and hobbies to explore, from art and nature to music and meeting new people. However, if food is our preoccupation and our primary source of delight, we will miss out on the other interesting aspects of life.

Jesus said, "I am the way and the truth and the life" (John 14:6). God will heal us because He doesn't want us operating in a system of lies. When we use food to help us deal with an unrelated issue, we are believing the lie that food is going to solve the problem. Psychologists refer to this unhelpful pattern as "indirectly coping." Rather than directly addressing a problem, we cope by overeating. Sometimes we do this because we know how to be upset with ourselves about our overeating, but we don't know how to be upset about or face the actual problem that led us to eat in the first place. Emotional eating pioneer Geneen Roth called this habit "shifting the drama." We are living a lie when we eat food to solve an unrelated problem or to soothe us when we are hurting. Isaiah 44:20 says, "Such a person feeds on ashes; a deluded heart misleads him; he cannot save himself, or say, 'Is not this thing in my right hand a lie?'" I hate to be the bearer of bad news, but this "thing in your right hand," the food, is a lie and will not save you or deliver you from the real issue underneath.

It's helpful to pause in a moment of stress or conflict and say, "This person is upsetting me, but I am not going to add calories to my body just because that person hurt my feelings." Adding calories to your body will never solve a problem with your friend. Furthermore, it's a lie to believe that God loves us or thinks we are "good" based on how we eat or what we look like. If we try to eat a certain way or be thin (which can lead to rebound bingeing), we are operating under the misconception that God's love for us is affected by how we eat or what we look like. These are lies, I tell you, and they remind me of that famous scene in the movie *Elf*, when Buddy the Elf told Santa he "sat on a throne of lies." God wants His daughters to live in the truth.

Finally, expect healing because God is a healer—it's who He is and what He does. When the Israelites came out of captivity in Egypt, God told them, "I am the LORD, who heals you" (Exodus 15:26). Just as the sun's nature is to shine and bring warmth and energy to our planet, God's inherent nature is to be our healer. When we are healed and know to give God the credit, He is glorified. We tell others how He set us free, which leads them to go to God for healing, creating intimacy between them and God.

THE HEALING PROCESS

Let's now look at *how* God heals us. Just like the dilapidated house, it's an inside-out transformation. Others may not see the change right away. Jesus said in Matthew 23:25–26, "Woe to you, teachers of the law and Pharisees, you hypocrites! You clean the outside of the cup and dish, but inside they are full of greed and self-indulgence. Blind Pharisee! First clean the inside of the cup and dish, and then the outside also will be clean."

The problem with diets is that they only address the outside of the cup. Diet gurus are not interested in the inside of your cup, and they certainly make more money if they can keep you focused on your cup's exterior without dealing with the invisible reasons leading you to overeat. They know that by solely treating the surface behaviors of how much you eat and what types of food you eat, you'll never address the underlying reasons for your destructive habit. You won't be completely healed in the way that brings permanent change, which means you'll keep circling back to fad diets, which keeps money in their pockets. I don't know about you, but I want permanent freedom in this area—I need to move on with my life! I assume that you also have better things to do with your time than think about food and your body until you die.

Let's seek healing the way Jesus recommends. If you start with your heart's feelings and your mind's thoughts (together, the inside of your cup), God can help you experience change in how you think and feel about food. As your thoughts and feelings change, your behavior (the outside of your cup) often follows. This "cognitive-behavioral approach," or influencing the mind to affect a person's behavior, has become a common practice in the field of psychology since it was developed by the psychiatrist Dr. Aaron Beck in the 1960s.

However, centuries before the cognitive-behavioral approach was conceived or supported by numerous research trials, the apostle Paul wrote to the Romans, "Do not conform any longer to the pattern of this world, but be transformed by the renewing of your mind. Then you will be able to test and approve what God's will is—his good, pleasing and perfect will" (Romans 12:2). Jesus communicated a similar idea when He said, "For the mouth speaks what the heart is full of" (Matthew 12:34). What you say and do are by-products of your heart's condition. The tongue is only a muscle that speaks what the heart and mind produce. Therefore, what's inside your heart affects how you speak. I would argue that, out of the emptiness of our hearts, the mouth also eats! When we explore the terrain of our hearts and minds and pinpoint what leads us to overeat, the healing process has begun. Graduates of the Releasity course report that they now give more constructive thought to their eating than before. This change, which begins in the heart and mind, results in altered eating behavior.

Just like the old house I'd pass on my way to work, God slowly begins replacing old patterns with new ones. As we quiet ourselves to be still with God and pour out our honest feelings and thoughts to Him (not inviting our smartphones to join us), He will respond and show us what we are avoiding or hoping for when we overeat. We can sit quietly and wait for Scripture, ideas, words, or pictures of response. We can read our Bibles to know what God has to tell us about Himself, about us, and about our situation.

LEARNING TO LISTEN

Some of us need a significant transformation when it comes to seeing God for who He says He is rather than who we believe Him to be. One day on a hike, I poured out my honest feelings to Him, then waited in silence. I looked out over the mountain view and heard a spontaneous, internal, and interrupting voice remind me of Scripture: "I'm not who you say I am—I Am Who I Am" (Exodus 3:14). God wanted me to understand that I don't get to declare what His character is like. Instead, He accurately and consistently informs me of His nature.

One way He does this is through Scripture, such as in the Book of Psalms, where we find many examples of God's character. Psalm 103:8–14 says,

> The Lord is **compassionate and gracious, slow to anger, abounding in love**. He will not always accuse, nor will he harbor his anger forever; he does not treat us as our sins deserve or repay us according to our iniquities. For as high as the heavens are above the earth, so **great is his love** for those who fear him; as far as the east is from the west, so far has **he removed our transgressions from us**. As a father has compassion on his children, so **the Lord has compassion** on those who fear him; for he knows how we are formed, he remembers that we are dust.

If we do not see God as He defines Himself, we must spend time being honest about who we erroneously believe Him to be. We must reorient our view of God in a way that agrees with what He says about Himself in the Bible. Pondering these truths reminds us of His love and kindness toward us.

In the coming week, spend time meditating on the different aspects of God's character as described in Psalm 103. Additional passages are included in the back of this book to help you further explore who God says He is. When we believe in and receive God's love toward us, we begin to trust Him and are more likely to seek His guidance with how to eat in a way that is beneficial to our bodies. This helps us not be controlled by the world's diet rules or our own excessive eating.

During the first year that I ran the Releasity course, I woke up one morning and felt compelled to grab a pen and write down a message. I'd never had this experience before, feeling like an invisible God was prompting me to do something so quickly and specifically. I looked around my disorganized bedside table to find the closest writing tool and a piece of scrap paper. Then the words came: *Tell them I love them. That it breaks my heart when they go to food instead of me. It will never satisfy—it will never be enough. Taste of my greatness and goodness, my tender care, my mercy. I'm not angry—I only want you to come to me.*

I immediately knew these words were a message from God for the women going through the Releasity course. I'm also sure they are words for you as you read this book today and take the steps of Releasity.

Another exchange takes place as we receive God's love. Because God sees us as valuable, we begin to agree with Him and show love and kindness to ourselves. We align our thoughts with what God says is true about us, and we gain an accurate perspective of ourselves. As Dr. Lou Priolo, a biblical counselor, writes, "When a Christian evaluates himself (as every person does continually), it is important for him to evaluate himself accurately. An accurate self-perception involves a clear understanding not only of what is wrong and needs to be corrected, but also of what is right and pleasing to God."[2] The back of this book also contains various Scriptures to read in order to gain an accurate understanding of who God says we are. Take some time to explore those verses and write down what God says is true about you. Some women are uncomfortable saying positive things about themselves or even receiving compliments with a simple "thank you." I'm not asking you to be arrogant about yourself, just accurate.

As we receive God's love and let it sink in, we are transformed into knowing our worth comes from what God says about us.

Rediscovering God's kindness toward us leads us to consider what the Bible says is good and true of us. We then begin to be "curious and not critical" toward ourselves. I paid thousands of dollars in counseling fees, and it was worth it just to learn this one phrase. When you are "curious and not critical," you ask yourself why you are overeating. This means saying something like, "Hmm, I wonder why I just ate an entire sleeve of Ritz crackers?" instead of beating yourself up and saying, "I did it again. I'll never have self-control. I'll never get it together. I'm a terrible person." Gently ask questions about your habits, rather than harming yourself with shameful thoughts and words. Through this practice, you build awareness of your motives and thoughts around stress and overeating.

If you liked that phrase, I've got another helpful one for you: "kinder is faster." If we will be kind to ourselves when we fail, we will not lose time and progress having to recover from the unkind words we are accustomed to brandishing toward ourselves. We begin to agree with God and echo the words in Psalms 139:14: "I praise you because I am fearfully and wonderfully made." We stop believing the world's lies about all the ways we don't measure up when it comes to our bodies and our beauty. We stop believing the hurtful messages of the people in our lives who have harmed us with unkind words.

Ultimately, God begins to replace our old habits with new ones, and our behaviors change. We used to turn to food when trying to cope with unrelated problems, but God sets us on a new path He has designed. As we let God into our hearts and allow Him to transform our minds, we discover that we don't follow the old patterns in a way that automatically connects our pain to food. Anna, a Releasity participant, shared that years after finishing the class, she still doesn't overeat because she just doesn't like to feel stuffed. This was new for her. An old proverb warns us to "go often to the house of a friend for weeds choke the unused path." When we turn to God for comfort, we abandon the faulty trail that connected our pain to the pantry. Our hearts rest where they were intended to find true intimacy, with God.

Our desires also begin to change through a peculiar and wonderful transformation. After receiving God's love toward us and showing ourselves love, we no longer desire excess food like we once did. Amanda, another Releasity graduate, shared how her husband suggested they get donuts in the afternoon after they'd already eaten cinnamon rolls earlier in the day. After completing Releasity, she knew doubling down on sweets was not a good idea and reminded him they had already had cinnamon rolls that morning. But a year before taking the class, it wouldn't have occurred to her that two treats in one day was unusual. This marked a new path for her mind to take, one that God was in the process of restoring.

Because we are learning how we have used food to cope with a non-food issue (like work or marriage stress), we begin to recognize the lie of thinking food will help us. We are changed in that we don't want to add weight to our body just because someone hurt our feelings or because we are stressed or bored. We begin to go to God for comfort and soothing and find other life-giving activities to relieve stress and pass the time until we feel physical hunger again. We no longer see excess eating as a viable recreational activity or source of entertainment. We are getting healthy! We know God loves us and we can trust His wisdom and guidance to eat "just enough" (Proverbs 25:16) as we follow His guidelines on the amount of food that is sufficient for us. We begin to like ourselves and want to do good things for ourselves. It's truly a miracle of God's healing.

I became aware of this transformation in my own life when my daughter was dedicated as an infant in our church. Prior to that time, I sometimes scoured the pantry to find enough food to cope with my unsettling emotions, but something different happened as I nervously anticipated her dedication. My husband and I had invited some family and friends to join us for the occasion, and I began to feel anxious and insecure about what our extended family would think about our rather "lively" church, which was so different from the church I grew up in. After getting ready for the service and realizing I had a few minutes to spare before we needed to leave, I told my husband I was going for a short stroll. I walked the sidewalk around our neighborhood that was lined with condos built in the 1940s. Pulling my cream-colored peacoat around me for warmth, it suddenly occurred to me that I had chosen to walk and pray to calm myself, rather than putting food in my mouth for relief from my emotions. Ten years earlier, I would have headed to the kitchen to deal with my anxiety, but God had changed my mind, heart, and will. I was now taking a route that pleased Him, talking to Him and moving my body, rather than indulging in extra food that couldn't help me and may have even hurt me in the long run. As I walked and prayed, I was shocked, thrilled, and grateful that God had changed my desires.

Even though God brings about this life-giving transformation, we also have a responsibility. Just like Noah co-labored with God to build an ark, it's your turn to map out a new path with God. For me to witness the transformation in my student's dilapidated house, I had to actually make an effort to walk to the house, enter it, and experience the transformation.

EXPECT THE LORD TO HEAL

RECEIVING GOD'S LOVE

So what are your responsibilities in expecting the Lord to heal? First, **be honest about any lies you believe about God**. You won't surprise Him when you tell Him what you think. In fact, He already knows. People can feel distant from God or have a distorted view of Him for many reasons. You may have memories of painful church experiences, deep traumas, or abuse that you believe God allowed to happen to you or someone else. Perhaps you lost a loved one, or someone you love has a debilitating illness; perhaps you are the one with the illness. You may carry confusing guilt because of surviving when a loved one lost their life. You must also honestly examine whether your circumstances or earthly experiences with a father, mother, teacher, spiritual leader, or other authority figure have negatively shaped how you perceive God.

In my case, negative experiences with male authority figures led me to think of God as described in the Old Testament. But the original Hebrew word for the Holy Spirit is actually a feminine noun. Perhaps thinking of females who have shown you God's love can give you a more accurate glimpse of your loving heavenly father.

Next, we begin to focus on **receiving God's love.** Psalm 103:2 instructs us to "forget not all his benefits." We do this by devoting time each day to prayer and reading the Bible, in particular the verses about God's character. We can also intentionally experience God's kindness through others. Think of someone in your life who is kind to you or who has done something nice for you lately. A simple gesture can encourage our belief that God is good, and that His love moved through a person to show kindness toward us. Once, sitting at a staff meeting for my youth ministry job, I noticed my boss get up from the table to make some coffee for himself. He knew I liked coffee, too. To my surprise, when he returned to the table, he had prepared a mug for me as well! I thought of how his gesture reflected God's kindness toward me because God's love moved through him to show me kindness. God will always be kinder than the kindest human.

We also have a responsibility to be **gentle toward ourselves**. In my early days of therapy with Patti, I spent an entire session unknowingly saying all kinds of harsh words about myself. At the end, I learned she had been secretly keeping a list of all these self-directed negative comments. She read the list aloud to me, and I was disturbed, to put it mildly. I'd never dream of saying these words about anyone else, yet I'd declared them about myself. From that day forward, I made a commitment to not criticize myself or my body out loud, other than confessing genuine sin or admitting my mistakes or general weaknesses. I don't allow my daughters to do this either, and I try to help them see where the culture has caused women to relentlessly criticize themselves. Putting a stop to speaking these unkind and unhelpful words and committing to "never say negative" words about my body has been a key component in God healing me of body shame. Be gentle with yourself and repeat these key phrases in your head:

- Never say negative.

- Be curious, not critical.

- Kinder is faster.

- Be accurate, not arrogant.

We must guard ourselves against the negative messages that are so pervasive in the culture around us. Years ago, a popular current-events website served as my home page. For many days, the site's most prominently displayed article was about the ten most beautiful women in the world, and guess what? My name did not make the list! I became more discouraged every time I opened my laptop and saw Angelina Jolie's picture pop up. Finally, I decided to change my home page altogether. Only then could I go back to focusing on the truth of what God says about me without that distraction. We weren't born to believe we aren't beautiful. The world's negative messages cause us to lose this confidence.

Think for a minute about a child you know who is confident about their skills, appearance, or mind. The world hasn't shut them down yet. My daughters were born with beautiful blue eyes, inherited from their grandfathers because neither my husband nor I have blue eyes. By age two, my youngest daughter had already grown accustomed to routinely receiving compliments about her eyes. Even strangers would say to her, "You have the most beautiful blue eyes!" We didn't realize this message was sinking in until her Sunday school teacher casually told another child in the class, "You have the most beautiful blue eyes!" My daughter immediately and confidently corrected the teacher by saying, "No, she doesn't. I do!" My daughter was beautiful, and she knew it!

So, you may be wondering, how long will all this transformation take? While God wants us to live in freedom and truth and by His nature wants to and *will* heal us so we can have more intimacy with Him, you may not see these changes overnight. We didn't get to our present state overnight, and God will likely not resolve it with a quick fix. Be thankful for that. If God condensed all the healing we need into a week's time frame, we'd be incredibly overwhelmed. We'd also miss out on all the insight the Holy Spirit gives when we approach healing by starting with the heart and mind. We gain intimacy with God through this process—and the process leads to a long-term solution. The lessons God will teach you are ones you will share with others for their benefit and God's glory.

Your transformation may also not be visible to others for a while. This isn't a quick "drop thirty pounds in two months" plan that attracts superficial compliments within a few weeks. But we don't seek the praise of people; we seek God's heart. He will keep guiding us. That being said, when I return to my hometown and see people I haven't seen in thirty years, I do hear compliments like, "You look amazing! You're half the person you used to be!" In these moments, I walk away and ponder the way God has healed me for the long-term by starting with the inside of my heart.

EXPECT THE LORD TO HEAL

REFLECTION QUESTIONS

Jot down the key ideas covered in this chapter.

What are some things you believed as a child but later realized were not actually true?

Early in the chapter, you were asked to rate your level of confidence that God could and would heal you of overeating (on a scale from 1 to 5). In the lines below, write the number you chose and why.

Three reasons were named for why God will heal us of overeating: so that we can be intimate with God, so that we can be free from bondage, and so that we can live in the truth. Which of these most appeals or relates to you?

What are some unhelpful thoughts or false perceptions you may have about God at this time?

_____

_____

_____

_____

If you feel distant from God at times, what are some reasons that you have felt this distance in those moments or seasons?

_____

_____

_____

_____

As we receive God's love for us, we begin to be kind toward ourselves. What are some ways you can show kindness toward yourself?

_____

_____

_____

_____

This chapter spoke of being "curious, not critical" toward ourselves when we eat in ways we regret. What are some "curious" and helpful questions you can ask yourself in moments when you feel like you have let yourself down?

_____

_____

_____

_____

EXPECT THE LORD TO HEAL

This chapter talked of the "inside-out transformation" that happens when we go to God for help with overeating. When have you experienced short-term weight loss from a diet that only addressed the "outside of the cup"? Why is it attractive and/or annoying to think of addressing the underlying causes of overeating in order to reach long-term weight loss?

_____

_____

_____

_____

As we form a new path of going to God instead of overeating, an "exchange" is taking place in our hearts. We see God differently, we see ourselves differently, and we begin to desire less food. As a step toward seeing yourself differently, write down one physical feature about yourself that you admire (for example, eyes, height, long fingers).

_____

_____

_____

_____

SET FREE & SATISFIED

JOURNALING

Set a timer for five minutes and write any thoughts, reflections, or new insights. You may want to write down any recent challenges or victories you have experienced related to your body, eating, or your emotions. Use the space below to write during the five minutes.

EXPECT THE LORD TO HEAL

MEMORIZE

Choose one of the following verses and write it on an index card or Post-it Note where you can see it each day. Try to say it out loud daily and commit it to memory during this week.

"Lord my God, I called to you for help, and you healed me."
—Psalm 30:2

"Praise the Lord, my soul, and forget not all his benefits—who forgives all your sins and heals all your diseases, who redeems your life from the pit and crowns you with love and compassion, who satisfies your desires with good things so that your youth is renewed like the eagle's."
—Psalm 103:2–5

Copy this verse in the space below as you begin to commit it to memory. If you choose a different verse, write it in the space below.

PRAYER

Check in with your friend who is supporting you in prayer. You may also want to write a prayer for yourself and post it where you can see it (and pray it!) each day, asking God to heal you in the area of overeating. Take a moment to write your own prayer to God in the space below.

_____

_____

_____

_____

_____

PRACTICE

Remember to show yourself love and self-care. Challenge yourself to not say any negative words out loud about your body. Invite a friend to join you and check in with each other after a few days to see how it's going. What are you noticing about your typical way of speaking about yourself? Are you curious or critical?

CHAPTER 4

Live Out of Your Freedom

I am no bird; and no net ensnares me; I am a free human being, with an independent will; which I now exert to leave you.
—Charlotte Bronte, *Jane Eyre*

Unless you've been living under a rock, you know there's an American fast-food restaurant that specializes in serving chicken sandwiches and waffle fries, and unfortunately for all of us, it's closed on Sundays. It's no misfortune for Chick-fil-A. Even though it operates one less day per week than its competitors, Chick-fil-A still ranked as the most popular fast-food restaurant in the United States in 2022 for the eighth year in a row.[1] The company's founder began shuttering the restaurants on Sundays as a religious decision, honoring God's command to rest on the Sabbath, and also to let his employees rest. But this happens to also be a brilliant business move. Why? Because of something economists and psychologists call the scarcity principle. It means that when we can't have something, demand for it increases. Monday through Saturday, people are subconsciously thinking, *I better get my Chick-fil-A because I won't be able to get it on Sunday!*

The scarcity principle is not only in effect when you can't have something but also when you *think* you can't have it. When it comes to the world's habit of dieting and following man-made food rules, we also appear to operate under this scarcity principle. We *believe* we "can't have" certain foods because they are "bad."

I once stood in a grocery-store checkout line and ran into an acquaintance waiting in front of me. As she and I made small talk, our conversation turned to the items in her cart. She began telling me about her latest diet and all the foods she "could have" and "couldn't have" on this program. All I could think was, *Who says you can't have it? Who's the person in charge of the diet that is currently ruling you?*

Another day, I was at a continuing-education conference for speech therapists when a group of people I didn't know invited me to join them for lunch. A woman I'd just met sat beside me and leaned in to scold me, saying, "You're being bad. You're drinking a Diet Coke!" Later that day, another woman saw me back at the conference, eating carrots for my snack, and said, "You're being good; you're eating carrots." It was dizzying! How did what I put in my mouth in a four-hour span determine the moral fabric of my character?

Are there foods you think you "can't have" or "shouldn't have," or foods that you call "bad," which just makes you want them all the more? For me, chocolate was once on all three of those lists. Poor chocolate! I thought I "couldn't have it," so I wanted it more. I obsessed over it and, in doing so, I allowed it to control me. While some foods have more nutrients than others, Jesus said, "What goes into someone's mouth does not defile them, but what comes out of their mouth, that is what defiles them" (Matthew 15:10). What you eat isn't the problem. It's what's in your heart that leads to the real problems of life.

Evelyn Tribole and Elyse Resch, authors of *Intuitive Eating,* an approach to eating with freedom, write that "if you tell yourself that you can't or shouldn't have a particular food, it can lead to intense feelings of deprivation that build into uncontrollable cravings and, often, bingeing. When you finally 'give-in' to your forbidden food, eating will be experienced with such intensity, it usually results in Last Supper overeating, and overwhelming guilt."[2] It turns out that having a "can't have" mindset with food is counterproductive.

To be set free from overeating, we must stop believing the world's message that there are foods we "can't have" and embrace the freedom God has given us. With this freedom, we can start making wise choices that are beneficial for our bodies. We begin to learn the meaning of 1 Corinthians 6:12: "'I have the right to do anything,' you say—but not everything is beneficial. 'I have the right to do anything'—but I will not be mastered by anything."

With that, it's time to talk about Step Three of Releasity: **Live Out of Your Freedom**. The previous two steps are to (R)emember What You Want and (E)xpect the Lord to Heal. When you embrace the third step and (L)ive Out of Your Freedom, you stop letting diets control you. You no longer crave excess food and don't want to rebel with food because you aren't restricting yourself by telling yourself you can't have something. You begin to enjoy your autonomy and learn how to make different choices with food using your God-given freedom. In this chapter, we will look at three components of eating with freedom: knowing the problem with diets, accepting the promise of freedom, and starting the process of approaching food in this new way.

So what's wrong with diets? Verses from Colossians help highlight their shortcomings. Paul, writing to a church about not being deceived and not following human rules says, "Therefore do not let anyone judge you by what you eat or drink" (Colossians 2:16). He continues in verses 20–23:

> Since you died with Christ to the elemental spiritual
> forces of this world, why, as though you still belonged to
> the world, do you submit to its rules: "Do not handle!
> Do not taste! Do not touch!"? These rules, which have
> to do with things that are all destined to perish with use,
> are based on merely human commands and teachings.
> Such regulations indeed have an appearance of wisdom,
> with their self-imposed worship, their false humility, and
> their harsh treatment of the body, *but they lack any value
> in restraining sensual indulgence* (italics mine).

The diet approach "lacks any value" for several reasons. First, diets make us dependent on something external to control us. God gave us free will at birth—and we were meant to grow up and learn how to be responsible and make good choices. Many of us missed this lesson. Some of us grew up overly controlled and largely managed by something outside of us—a controlling parent or a family who was primarily concerned with the image we portrayed to outsiders. Some of us were neglected as children and had no one guiding us toward responsible and wise choices. Perhaps we didn't have adults in our lives who modeled discipline. As a result, we have given power to other people in some areas of our lives and, for those of us who overeat, we are tempted to allow diets to tell us how to eat.

We shift responsibility and power to someone or something outside of us to make us behave—or even blame those external forces when we don't behave, like my former coworker who came into work one morning with a hangover, claiming he had been "overserved" the night before. In looking to diets to fix us, we deny our personal responsibility in making changes and ignore our own "inner voice" leading us. We don't listen to what we are feeling on the inside and don't develop maturity with our freedom. God doesn't want us to be dependent on something outside of us to make wise choices, but instead instructs us: "Do not be like the horse or the mule, which have no understanding but must be controlled by bit and bridle or they will not come to you" (Psalm 32:9).

Recently I saw this play out at a restaurant. I had finished eating my meal because I was physically satisfied and my friend said to me, "Weight Watchers says you can have as many fruits and veggies as you want. Keep eating!" But I wasn't hungry, so I told her, "Weight Watchers doesn't decide what I eat—I do!"

Second, diets don't have the power to change our desires or make us want less food. Diets are just words on paper. As the above verses from Colossians remind us, diets are not capable of restraining indulgence. Diets do not fix our way of eating; they are simply a standard against which we judge our eating. The diet itself has no power, but we sadly give it power over us. When we do so, we will ultimately rebel because we weren't meant to live under their control. If we accidentally break our diet rules at 4 p.m., we often take it as a license to binge eat the rest of the day. This is absurd because we wouldn't do this with anything other than food. Imagine discovering a small hole in your skirt, then deciding to rip up the rest of the skirt!

We need the power to make lasting change, and it won't come from diet instructions. The real solution is to have something or someone operating inside of us that actually has power to transform our desires and is supportive of our desire to eat a reasonable amount of food. God gave us the Holy Spirit to bring about this change as we connect with Him in the area of food. Releasity isn't about following a bunch of rules for how to eat. It's about maturing with your freedom and asking God to walk alongside you and empower you to make food choices that are beneficial to your body and overall lifestyle goals. You get to decide, with your freedom, what foods you want to choose. You can ask God to guide you, and He will.

My last hang-up with diets is that they often distract us mentally and keep God out of the process. When God is not the one teaching you how to eat in a beneficial way, something else will become your god. Either your diet or certain "healthy foods" will become your god, or attaining your desired weight will. We try to obey the food rules instead of obeying and following the one true God. This keeps us focused on dieting, food, and our bodies—sometimes to the point of obsession—and we don't think as much about loving God and loving other people, which is what Jesus said is the greatest command (Matthew 22:37–39).

Dining out with a friend one evening, the conversation veered from meaningful conversation about the current events in our lives and the world to my friend's latest attempts to manage her weight through intermittent fasting. As she talked on and on about tracking macros and introduced other vocabulary I didn't recognize, I thought, *She is thinking about this way too much!* All the focus on food content and dieting was distracting her from God. He would guide her if she would go to Him! Worse, when we have success apart from God, we risk becoming prideful and thinking we don't need God's help.

I made a great mistake in this area. During a season of significant weight loss, I took a walk with a friend along the Key Bridge in Washington, DC. As we looked over the Potomac River that divided Virginia from the Capitol Mall with its monuments and museums, she asked me, "Do you ever worry you'll gain the weight back?"

I ignorantly and now regretfully responded, "Oh, no! I don't go up on the scale. My weight only goes down on the scale." Let's just say that was a short-sighted and ignorant answer. After restricting my eating, losing weight, and then becoming prideful because of my short-lived dieting success, I actually began to rebound and binge, not relying on God to guide my eating. Just as God's Word says that "pride goes before destruction, a haughty spirit before a fall" (Proverbs 16:18), my disordered binge eating picked up soon after that walk and I learned how prideful I had become, trying to lose weight apart from God. My friend Danielle posed the following question to me after thinking through this idea: "Would you rather get to your ideal weight and be arrogant and distant from God, or get to your ideal weight and be humble, thankful, and reliant on God?" I'd choose the latter.

THE PROMISE OF FREEDOM

Maybe you aren't convinced that living out of your freedom is a more powerful option than following diet rules. Maybe you don't believe me when I say that God wants you to understand the autonomy you have when it comes to food. For this reason, we must talk about God's "promise of freedom."

First and simply, you were born free—all children come out of their mother's womb with the independence to cry and scream at the top of their lungs. Most do, trust me, and they don't stop for a while.

Older children may choose to obey but still express themselves in other ways, such as the rowdy boy in Sunday school whose teacher instructed him to sit down. After he reluctantly sat, he called out to his teacher, "I may be sitting on the outside, but I am standing on the inside!" Similarly, you have the right and ability to put this book down and head to your local grocery store just to buy your favorite treat because you are likely an adult with car keys and a wallet. No one, not even God, is stopping you.

Second, you are free to eat because eating however you please does not jeopardize God's love for you. God loves you no matter how or what you eat, no matter how much you weigh, and no matter what you look like. You simply cannot lose His love. Romans 8:38 says, "For I am convinced that neither death nor life, neither angels nor demons, neither the present nor the future, nor any powers, neither height nor depth, nor anything else in all creation, will be able to separate us from the love of God that is in Christ Jesus." I'm not sure of any simpler way to say this: You cannot lose God's love. The way you eat does not separate you from His love.

The first church my young family attended often reminded the children, "God loves you, no matter what!" I realized this message was sinking in when I sent my three-year-old daughter to her room for a disciplinary time-out. As she hesitantly but obediently went to her room, she looked back and made sure to remind me with a shout, "Well, God still loves me, no matter what!"

The same is true for you—and it gets better. Your righteousness before God (which means being "right with God" or appearing blameless before God) doesn't depend on what you weigh, how you eat, or what you look like. Your righteousness with God is based on what Jesus did on the cross for you two thousand years ago. He died on the cross and "bore the sin of many," according to Isaiah 53:12.

Why did he bear your sin on his body in this mysterious way? Because we have a perfect, loving God who wants to be in relationship with us. However, because of our imperfect nature, or sins, God is unable to be in our presence and remain holy. Just like a bride's perfect white wedding dress would be sullied by a muddy dog running up to it, interacting with our sin would make God impure. Something must be done to remove our sin, which is why God sent Jesus to shed His blood on the cross. In doing so, Jesus bore the punishment of our sins and cleansed us of our iniquities. We are now able to be in God's holy presence. We are made righteous in God's eyes because of what Jesus did for us, not because of any way we behave on earth, including how we eat.

When we trust in what Jesus did for us and put our faith in Him, we have what is called "passive righteousness." This means we don't do a thing to be righteous before God. Rather, we simply receive what Jesus did for us through faith. We don't have to perform a certain way or look a certain way to be "right" or *eat* a certain way to be right.

However, many Christians miss out on the rest and joy that come from this passive righteousness. Instead, we try to be righteous on our own. This is called "active righteousness," or "works-based theology." We may think we are good at certain things and feel good about ourselves because we consider ourselves smarter, more generous, or more humble than the next person, for example. Oddly enough, when I first learned of this concept, I realized that I found some of my righteousness in being a good speller. It probably sounds silly to you, but on some days, if I blew it in one area of life, I felt better knowing I could still take pride in my spelling (which is something I inherited genetically, I admit, and most people don't care how well you spell!).

We believe we are pleasing God through our works, but the Bible teaches that "our righteous acts are like filthy rags" to God (Isaiah 64:6). Any kind of righteousness we try to attain apart from Jesus making us pure and righteous through bearing our sins on the cross does not measure up and won't give us true peace. Jesus died so we wouldn't have to follow rules to be righteous. When we live under food or diet rules, we are not living the way God intended. Galatians 5:1 says, "It is for freedom that Christ has set us free. Stand firm, then, and do not let yourselves be burdened again by a yoke of slavery."

By dying on the cross, Jesus paid the penalty for every sin we ever committed or ever will commit, and we aren't under the Old Testament law where we have to keep rules. Therefore, all things are *permissible,* "but not everything is beneficial" (1 Corinthians 6:12). Furthermore, "There is now no condemnation for those who are in Christ Jesus" (Romans 8:1). We are not in trouble with God for how we eat! Overeating or gluttony is not a salvation deal-breaker. If you are trusting in what Jesus did on the cross to make you righteous, you do not trust in how you eat or how you care for your body or what you look like to be right before God.

THE PROCESS OF FREEDOM

That all sounds good, right? But how do you make this a reality in your life? First, I encourage you to eat whatever kinds of foods you want because you know you are free to have them. Think about your "can't have, shouldn't have, or bad" foods and see if there are some you'd really like to eat. Begin to eat them as a normal part of your day, at a mealtime or as a snack. You may be hesitant to try this approach because you've never known how to be responsible with food, but hang on with me for a second. Remember, the food going into your body isn't morally good or bad. Recall what Jesus said, that it isn't what goes in your mouth that makes you clean or unclean (Matthew 15:11). Also, this "freedom" approach is supported by research. Treatment methods related to "food habituation" and "cue exposure" have been proven to reduce the overeating of foods that were previously eaten in excess. It turns out that if you give yourself freedom and regular access to the foods that typically lead to binge eating, you are more likely to lose the desire to eat those foods in excess.[3]

When we begin to enjoy foods we thought were forbidden, we mentally remind ourselves, "God still loves me. I'm not in trouble for eating this." We can relax, knowing that freedom means no longer hiding junk food in drawers or sneaking through the fast-food drive-thrus. You don't have to hide in a dark car with a package of Oreos and a carton of milk, like I did during my disordered eating days. We begin to exercise our freedom to eat anything, knowing we cannot lose God's love for us, no matter what. We absorb the fact that being "right with God" has nothing to do with how we look or what we eat. Jesus died to make us righteous; we don't diet to be made righteous.

A couple of caveats should be addressed as you try out your freedom with foods. Please don't eat something to which you have a known allergy; be wise and responsible in that regard. Second, if you are thinking, *I eat what I want anyway, so why is this different?*, is it possible that you eat it because you think you can't have it or that it's forbidden? Your shift will need to be in what you tell yourself as you are enjoying the food. Instead of thinking, *I'm doing something I shouldn't be doing*, remind yourself, *I'm not breaking a rule; I have freedom because Jesus said it's not what goes in me that makes me unclean.* Remind yourself that how you eat doesn't affect God's love for you or your salvation. The Releasity approach starts with freedom. We were meant to ask God to guide us to make wise and beneficial choices with that freedom. As you use this autonomy to make beneficial choices with food, I imagine you'll see other areas of your life where your ability to choose makes a positive difference.

Once we begin to understand that we have options, it's amazing how we start to think straight and aren't desperate for food all the time. We can be honest about what we want. We know we are free to eat four pieces of pizza because eating a certain way doesn't make us righteous, but a strange, new thought enters: *Wait, I actually don't want four pieces of pizza. What I really want is sleep!* Now that we aren't eating out of deprivation, rebound, or rebellion, we begin to detect a form of wisdom bubbling up inside. We continue to be curious and ask ourselves questions like, *Do I even like the food I'm eating? Am I tired? Do I need sleep? Am I eating because I feel guilty for not calling my mom? Do I feel sad that I can't call my mom?* We also might ask ourselves if we are physically hungry in that moment. We may start to think in terms of using our freedom to choose foods that are beneficial to our bodies and offer us nutritional value (what I call "Maker-made" foods, ones that come from plants). We might use our freedom to add a salad to our day. We can even use our freedom to say, "Instead of eating about my stress, I'm going to take a walk or call a friend."

Now that we are experimenting with this new approach to food, we sense that God is leading us to learn wisdom in our food choices. We bring to mind all the new revelations or reminders we have about God loving us that we discovered during the last chapter. God is good and we can trust what He says. As we begin to trust God, through our inner voice, we begin hearing nudges of the Holy Spirit who is giving us instructions for when and how to eat. We begin to spend intentional time seeking God through prayer and we tune into His gentle guidance. We don't perfect this right away (or ever, because we are human), but we recognize our moments of overeating as a "check engine" light on our mental and emotional "dashboard," giving us clues as to what might be driving us to overeat. We can pray to God for help, rather than indirectly coping with our pain by going to food.

Tuning in to God's guidance through the Holy Spirit reminds me of alcoholics who meet a sponsor through their twelve-step recovery program. In the same way they communicate with one person who has been through the program before them, we can meet with the Holy Spirit for companionship and guidance with food. This ongoing communication with God as we process our eating habits becomes an intimate dance with God. We don't want to miss the beauty and joy of it! Isaiah 30:21 says, "Your ears will hear a voice behind you saying, 'This is the way; walk in it.'" We no longer have to stick to a certain diet that we will inevitably fail to keep, but we can ask the Spirit to give us wisdom and help to develop a plan with our freedom. As the Holy Spirit gives us direction, we don't always have to think about what we will eat next.

There are many ways to be careful with our eating, but I find that initially writing down my feelings or food choices on a daily basis helps me reflect on my eating habits. I can then think about whether or not I want to make those same choices again in the future. If a plan to keep track of your eating and your feelings is helpful, remember that this is a *tool, not a rule*! Continue to be curious about how you feel after eating certain foods or amounts of food. Don't criticize yourself for your less healthy food choices; know that you chose to eat that way in freedom. Be flexible and be a learner. You can look at a day's eating and think, *What might I want to change tomorrow?* instead of, *What do I have to change?* Ask yourself, *What do I choose to eat with my freedom?* instead of, *How much can I get away with eating?* It's no longer an issue of what food you can or can't have. The question instead becomes: *What and how do I choose to eat with my freedom?* It's choice-based, not rules-based.

We ask God to grow wisdom in us and give us the grace of self-control with food as we learn how to eat freely in a way that doesn't cause harm to our bodies or eventually lead to health problems. Proverbs 24:13–14 says, "Eat honey, my son, for it is good; honey from the comb is sweet to your taste. Know also that wisdom is like honey for you: If you find it, there is a future hope for you, and your hope will not be cut off." We receive God's love, trust Him, love ourselves, and show Him our love by trying to follow His guidance.

During one of my counseling sessions with Patti, the crux of our discussion was a Twix candy bar that had been sitting in the window-sill just over my kitchen sink at home. At this point, I shared a house with two new roommates, and we had a friend who was a resident in medical school. He'd often stop by and visit us after his long shifts at the hospital. Marty enjoyed bringing us gifts and had dropped off a Twix bar someone had given him at the hospital. I was both fixated on this Twix bar and furious, because I wanted to eat it, but I also didn't want to eat it. He'd left it for us to be nice, but it was only a distracting and maddening temptation for me. Patti and I spent the hour in counseling talking about the Twix bar, which was controlling me because it was at that time one of my "can't have" foods. I had obsessed over fighting to have self-control and not eat that candy bar because I knew it was forbidden to me.

After I explained my dilemma, Patti gently asked, "I'm sorry, I don't understand. Why can't you eat the Twix bar?"

I looked out the window of her office and tried to verbalize my still cloudy thought process. "I guess I think that if I eat that Twix bar, I'll never lose the weight I need to lose in order to be thin enough to have a man be attracted to me and then to marry me."

With a hint of playful sarcasm, Patti responded, "Oh, I get it . . . if you eat that Twix bar, you are never going to get married. I don't blame you. I wouldn't eat it either!"

I recognized the absurdity of what she was saying, which was just a synthesis of what I'd verbally unearthed from my psyche. I then realized I had given this Twix bar too much power over me and my entire life trajectory. She then began to talk about my freedom, and how my "trigger foods" had gained power over me because I thought they were forbidden.

Patti encouraged me to take a week to eat the foods I thought were forbidden, remembering that God loved me no matter what food I ate. I left her office and drove straight to the grocery store. My first stop was the frozen-food aisle, where I bought a box of the Toaster Strudel pastries I had enjoyed in my lonely years as a latchkey kid. It felt incredible and foreign to "try on" this freedom!

I realize this step involves trust and trying something new. Please give yourself permission to be in a state of growing and learning; finding your freedom with food is a process. Even if your physician has recommended certain food choices, she is not tying you down and making you eat that way. Instead, hopefully you will use your freedom and wisdom to make beneficial choices as time goes on. Restrictive diets usually make us want the food more, like wanting Chick-fil-A because we can't have it on Sundays. God has given us freedom and He gave us food for pleasure. So many places in the Bible talk about food offerings being "pleasing aromas" to God. Eating one piece of chocolate cake when we celebrate with friends is pleasurable, but when we shove down four pieces of cake on a random Tuesday afternoon, we probably won't be as happy about how we've used our freedom! It's so important that we don't believe certain foods are being restricted. We choose what we want to eat or not eat. We are not afraid and do not need to feel like we will be in trouble if we eat a certain food. We can experience a delightful freedom to have as much or as little as we want.

REFLECTION QUESTIONS

Jot down a brief summary of the ideas shared in this chapter.

_____

_____

_____

_____

Name some foods you have previously considered to be "bad" or foods you have believed that you "couldn't have."

_____

_____

_____

_____

What are some foods you have considered as "good" or that you "can have"?

_____

_____

_____

_____

What are some other "food rules" you may have followed in the past that may not be from God?

_____

_____

_____

_____

This chapter mentioned a few shortcomings of diets. They included: relying on something outside of us to make us "behave," the fact that diets lack the power to change our desire to overeat, and that diets can leave God out of the process. What are some ways you have experienced any of these limitations in your own life through dieting?

———————————————————————————

———————————————————————————

———————————————————————————

———————————————————————————

What are some attractive reasons to rely on something outside of us to manage our eating habits?

———————————————————————————

———————————————————————————

———————————————————————————

———————————————————————————

Three reasons were given for why we have freedom to eat as we want: being born with a free will, not being able to lose God's love because of how we eat, and the fact that Jesus's death on the cross makes us "right" in the eyes of God (not how we eat, what we weigh, or what we look like). How is this different from what you have understood about eating in the past? What are your thoughts about this new way of approaching food with freedom and faith?

———————————————————————————

———————————————————————————

———————————————————————————

What are some foods that you've previously considered forbidden that you'd like to eat with freedom this week?

_____

_____

_____

_____

JOURNALING

Set a timer for five minutes and use the space below to write any new insights, thoughts, or reflections you had after reading this chapter. You can also use this space to write about recent victories or struggles related to your eating or your emotions.

_____

_____

_____

_____

_____

_____

_____

_____

_____

_____

_____

_____

_____

_____

_____

_____

_____

_____

_____

_____

_____

_____

_____

_____

_____

_____

MEMORIZE

Write the following verse on an index card where you can see it each day. Try to say it out loud daily and commit it to memory over the next week.

"It is for freedom that Christ has set us free. Stand firm, then, and do not let yourselves be burdened again by a yoke of slavery."
—Galatians 5:1

Write the verse in the space below as a way of beginning to memorize the verse.

_____

_____

_____

PRAYER

Continue to check in with your friend who is praying for you on this journey. Use the space below to write a prayer to God as you connect with Him in this area of your life.

PRACTICE

Remember to show yourself love and self-care. If you've never asked God to make you right and pure through what Jesus did for you on the cross, I pray you will explore this in the coming days and weeks. Talk with a trusted friend who is a Christian to understand more or seek out a church to have a conversation about what this means. The Bible says, "All have sinned and fall short of the glory of God" (Romans 3:23). It also says, "God demonstrates his own love for us in this: While we were still sinners, Christ died for us" (Romans 5:8).

It's a spiritual mystery, but the Bible teaches that the blood Jesus shed for us on the cross two thousand years ago in the Middle East makes us pure before a holy God. This enables us to be in God's presence, free from shame or condemnation. Romans 5:10–11 states, "For if, while we were God's enemies, we were reconciled to him through the death of his Son, how much more, having been reconciled, shall we be saved through his life! Not only is this so, but we also boast in God through our Lord Jesus Christ, through whom we have now received reconciliation." My prayer for you is that you will ask Jesus to be your Lord and Savior in His timing.

Practice living out of your freedom with food this week by eating foods you actually want to eat. Tell yourself as you eat, "God still loves me. I'm not in trouble. This food isn't 'bad.'" Receive God's love as you eat because you cannot lose His love. It is Jesus's death on the cross that makes you worthy, significant, and right before God, not what or how you eat. Take time to write and reflect on how it feels to eat foods that you had previously considered "forbidden."

CHAPTER 5

Eat with Hunger When You Feel It

*If you find honey, eat just enough—too much of it,
and you will vomit.*
—Proverbs 25:16

My mom's diesel Cadillac backed out of our driveway one chilly fall evening, and I couldn't believe my good fortune. There I was, a bright-eyed ten-year-old, sitting in the middle of the front seat, long before laws required kids to sit in the back or wear seatbelts. The occasion was my sister's sixteenth birthday, and my mom was treating her and three friends to dinner in the big city of Charlotte, an hour's drive from our rural home. I was thrilled to tag along, though I'm sure it wasn't my sister's first choice to have me there with her friends. They found good use for me, though, tasking me with switching the radio station whenever they tired of the song playing.

On both the way to dinner and the way home, I noticed there was one song the girls always wanted to hear. A woman named Madonna was singing about being "like a virgin," whatever that was, and she mentioned making it through the wilderness. The lyrics were catchy but odd to me, and after two hours in the car, I became quite familiar with the chorus.

When we returned home after dinner, my dad and brother joined us for birthday cake and ice cream. With all eight of us still gathered in our dining room, I noticed some increasing discomfort in my stomach region, having eaten the birthday dessert on top of my already massive restaurant meal. Feeling cool for having spent the evening with four teenage girls, I wanted to impress them with a joke. I made sure the room was completely quiet before delivering my line. Seizing the moment, I dramatically leaned forward to grab their attention. After contorting my face and placing my hands on my overly full belly, I moaned: "Ohhh! I feel like a virgin!" The room quickly erupted in shocked, hysterical laughter. I was absolutely confused and didn't get the amused and delighted response I wanted. Later, I learned what a virgin really was, as well as how to use (or not use) this new vocabulary word going forward.

That night sums up my younger self's cluelessness about what it felt like to be full after eating a great deal of food. I had no idea that humans are born with hunger and fullness cues within our bodies that help us know both when to eat and when to take a break from eating. It would be years before I came to understand how God designed this internal hunger system to guide us so we can enjoy food for both pleasure and nutrition.

We are now ready to move to Step Four of Releasity: **Eat with Hunger When You Feel It.** If you use this internal cueing system, eating inside your "hunger and fullness window," you will likely reach your healthy or ideal weight. **This is also where you begin to implement HELP, the acronym for how to keep a daily rhythm of following God's plan for your eating. The "H" stands for "hunger" and reminds you to wait for hunger before you eat.**

I wonder what your experience is with feeling hunger and knowing how to recognize it and let it guide you? Perhaps you're like me and your family simply ate meals and snacks according to the clock with no discussion of whether you were hungry or not. Breakfast was at seven o'clock, lunch at noon, a snack at three, and dinner at six. Never mind if it was Thanksgiving and you'd eaten two plates' worth of food at lunch, then grazed all afternoon on pies, cookies, and candy. Family dinner would still be promptly served at six o'clock!

It's helpful to pause and talk about what hunger even *is*. In the old days, before human physiology was understood, people recognized hunger as a sensation near our midline that told our minds we were out of food and needed more. It's similar to the feeling when your bladder lets you know you've had your fill of liquid and need to go to the bathroom. Just as pressure in the pelvic area signals that it's time to relieve yourself, a gnawing sensation in the stomach is your signal to go to the kitchen and eat.

Living in the twenty-first century, however, scientific advancements have identified the specific process occurring inside the human body when you feel hunger or fullness. As for hunger, we now know that after you eat a reasonable amount of food, your blood sugar (or the amount of glucose present in your blood) rises to a certain level. Later, once your body has used up the amount of food you ate, your blood sugar levels begin to drop, stimulating a hormone called ghrelin. Ghrelin's function is to let the brain (specifically, a part of the brain called the hypothalamus, which regulates some of your most basic body functions like sleep, thirst, and hunger) know that more food is needed. When the hypothalamus gets this message, it releases neuropeptides, which are neurotransmitters that stimulate your appetite. Essentially, they tell the stomach to start producing hydrochloric acid, which produces the empty growls or hollow, burning sensation that help you know your body is ready to eat more food.

As for fullness cues, your body registers these in two different ways from two different locations. When you feel the sensation of fullness, it is because your stomach wall has stretched, and nerve cells have relayed this message to the brain. Second, in a slower process, your gut registers the nutrient content of what you've eaten, and it generates other hormones that transmit the fullness message to the brain.

No matter how simply or sophisticatedly you describe it, an "intelligent designer" created us to have a stable, balanced state when it comes to hunger and satisfaction. It is amazing to consider that we have multiple body systems and that two of them—the nervous system and the digestive system—primarily communicate to help us know when to eat and when to stop. This simple "message system" of internal cues is God's way of guiding us with our eating. Learning to follow these cues is what enables us to enjoy food without gluttony and to recognize when we are using food for emotional comfort versus physical sustenance. It also helps us begin eating in a balanced way that leaves us at our ideal weight.

Please note that your ideal weight is likely *not* that of Twiggy, the super-thin supermodel of the 1960s, nor is your ideal body the one you had when you were twelve (if you were even thin at that age—I personally wasn't thin at twelve!). Your ideal, or healthy, weight will more likely reflect the genetics of your family heritage than the pictures of uber-thin celebrities seen in magazines for decades. My family heritage is German, so I'm not going to look like a petite French woman.

FEELING YOUR HUNGER

If we have this effective, God-designed system inside us meant to help us know how much to eat and when, why don't we regularly follow its cues? Understanding why we are unaware or mistrustful of these cues can be the key to awakening our bodies and re-learning to eat when we are hungry and stop when we are satisfied. Quickly, let's consider why we don't wait for hunger before we eat.

Some of us simply didn't learn this approach to eating as kids. A Releasity participant shared that she grew up with three older brothers, and if she didn't grab plenty of food at the first offer, she might not get any by the time her brothers finished taking what they wanted. She certainly didn't pay attention to her hunger! When I was twenty-five, a friend gifted me a book that talked about how to wait for hunger before eating and how to connect with God instead of food while waiting to hear your stomach growl or feel physical hunger pangs before eating. This was a brand new concept for me! The idea that I could wait for the sensation of hunger prior to eating and lose weight in the process was incredible. I had always eaten the way we ate when I was growing up—by the clock! Though I'm thankful my mother provided food for me in a predictable rhythm, I've also benefited as an adult from learning what it means to eat according to my hunger.

Another reason we don't wait for physical hunger is that we've discovered how eating can make us feel better emotionally. Eating certain kinds of food releases dopamine, a brain chemical that promotes feelings of pleasure and satisfaction. Somewhere along the way, whether through trial and error or by observing someone else eating for comfort, we learned the magical connection between popping a treat in our mouths and gaining momentary relief from feeling uncomfortable, sad, lonely, or bored. It brings to mind a popular fast-food bakery that offers a sweet to anyone who's had a problem with their order, promising a "treat for your trouble."

For me, this habit of eating to handle emotions started when I was a child, and a therapist told me I'd been smart and resourceful to eat sweets when I felt lonely or bored—that these were good problem-solving skills. However, she reminded me, I was no longer a child who only had sweets to make me feel better, and she urged me to recognize the freedom and new resources I have as an adult. I now have car keys, she said, and can leave my house to meet my needs creatively, rather than resorting to what might have been my sole option as a child.

If you have a history of dieting and following restrictive eating plans, you have grown accustomed to ignoring your body's internal signals. Though we rarely see anyone find long-term freedom from food and weight issues through diets, we are drawn to their promises. Most diets suggest that our bodies cannot be trusted, and over time, ignoring our internal hunger and fullness cues in favor of restrictive diets can lead to significant problems. The authors of Intuitive Eating say that consistently denying ourselves and not following our hunger and fullness cues can lead to our "feeling ravenous, not being in touch with hunger, obsessing with food, eating too fast, gaining weight, and having our metabolism slow down to conserve energy." [1]

You also may have learned to ignore your body's hunger and fullness cues because someone made you "clean your plate" as a child, regardless of whether or not you felt hungry. You may have been told that children were starving in some part of the world and your eating habits had some relationship to theirs. Let me assure you, eating more than you physically need will not help those children get the food they need. A better option is to send them a financial donation to help pay for the food they might actually see.

Some of us have also avoided waiting for hunger because we fear being hungry and see it as an enemy that must be avoided at all costs. You might think, *If I don't get hungry, I won't want to overeat, and then I will lose weight.* We may have gained this faulty rationale through advertisements stating that if we take a certain pill, we can avoid hunger, and thus avoid overeating. Interestingly, most of us don't overeat because we feel physical hunger; we overeat for reasons that will be addressed in later chapters. A current Christian diet plan guarantees "not feeling hunger," but I wonder why that is considered a good thing. God gave us hunger as a tool to guide us. Why wouldn't we want to feel it?

Feeling our hunger is a gift from God because we know our loving, brilliant Creator gave us these cues to help guide us, in line with His biblical promises to guide us throughout our lives. God means for you to enjoy food within your body's hunger and fullness window. One study found that physical hunger actually increases the sensitivity of the taste receptors on our tongues.[2] As a friend once told me, "Hunger is the best seasoning!" We can appreciate feelings of physical hunger and anticipate them as a gift from God. Along with the other ways He guides us, we want to let Him be our guide in this area. Proverbs 3:5, Isaiah 30:21, and Psalms 25:12 are all wonderful Scriptures that tell of His desire to guide us.

HOW TO FOLLOW HUNGER CUES

Now that we've talked about *what* hunger and fullness cues are and the various reasons we may have avoided following them, let's explore *how* to follow this divine guidance inside us.

Since this will be new to most readers, start by asking God to help you. Pray for the ability to eat within your hunger and fullness window on two types of occasions each day. Pray "in the moment" of temptation and also "out of the moment" of temptation. Pray Proverbs 25:16, which says, "If you find honey, eat just enough—too much of it, and you will vomit." We start by praying that God will help us eat "just enough" during the day.

Pray also the words of God's promise to us in 1 Corinthians 10:13: "God is faithful; he will not let you be tempted beyond what you can bear. But when you are tempted, he will also provide a way out so that you can endure it." Pray that God would provide you with a way out of the temptation to eat more than "just enough," that you will recognize that "way out," and that you will take that way out when it comes. Sometimes I know I've had enough to eat and then my food just "happens" to spill on the floor. I know that's God giving me my "way out."

Praying about your ability to eat when you are hungry and stop when you are satisfied has two great outcomes: intimacy with God and insight into your faulty pattern with food. This rhythm of wanting food but waiting for hunger and talking to God while you wait becomes a dance of intimacy with God. It's rare and beautiful. In Psalm 81:10, God said, "I am the LORD your God, who brought you up out of Egypt. Open wide your mouth and I will fill it." Egypt represents your bondage to overeating, and God longs to free you from the chains of overeating, so go to Him in prayer about this matter often. God wants to fill you with Himself and many other gifts rather than have you be filled with excess food! This is not to say you must sit in your room and read the Bible every time you are tempted to eat more than you are hungry for; rather, God will meet you and comfort you, then give you ideas of other life-giving activities to help you pass the time until you are hungry again.

Beyond intimacy, God will give you insight into why you go to excess food. As you are "curious, not critical," God begins to reveal to you your pattern of feeling stressed or restless and how you have gotten into a rut of turning to food with your problems and not to God.

Perhaps you're thinking, *This is too much work. I'll only give up in this process.* It's normal to grow weary of just trying to lose weight on the surface. It's hardly inspiring. But what if your motivation was intimacy with God and gaining insight into the root of your problem with food so that this struggle would leave you for life? That can motivate!

Now that we've prayed, let's practice the process with three steps or phases.

1. Wait for physical hunger before eating.

2. Eat with physical hunger.

3. Stop eating when you are satisfied.

Remember, you are "living out of your freedom" and asking God to guide you to make beneficial choices for your body. Be "curious, not critical" as you practice. Remember that "kinder is faster," and that this process is based on the Holy Spirit's help, not self-help.

WAITING FOR PHYSICAL HUNGER
BEFORE YOU EAT

The next time you want to eat, stop and ask yourself this simple question: "Am I hungry?" If the answer isn't a clear "yes" or "no," take the next step and begin to rate your hunger. When you are just beginning to follow your hunger cues, a Hunger Fullness Scale can be a helpful tool in learning to describe your sensations of hunger and fullness. Search online for "hunger fullness scales," find one you like, and print a couple of copies so you can place one in your kitchen and the other in your purse or office. Alternatively, download an image of one to your phone (or screenshot and save it) so you always have it with you. Most scales rate "1" as painfully hungry and "10" as painfully overstuffed, with "5" being a neutral feeling. When you want to eat, try to quantify how much hunger you are feeling at the time. You may want to write down what time you begin to feel hunger pangs or when you hear your stomach growling to keep tabs on your hunger; then write down subsequent times the feeling of hunger might be growing stronger.

If you find you want to eat but aren't physically hungry yet, that's normal! The word "change" is going to help you here. Change your environment or your activity to avoid temptation while you wait for hunger. I've even been encouraged to find an activity that is "incompatible with eating" and keeps my fingers occupied while I wait for physical hunger, like gardening, playing an instrument, or painting my nails. Visit the Releasity website to watch humorous videos with tips on how to take "Drastic Measures," including how to shove leftover cake down the drain and how to handle the pressure of a Thanksgiving meal with the accompanying social expectation of overeating. You're also never too old to create and enjoy a reward chart where you can rack up a certain number of checks for passing by food when you aren't physically hungry. Think of a relaxing or fun reward that will motivate you to stay on track.

EATING WITH HUNGER

Now, it's time for the fun part! If you haven't grazed, you should start to feel hunger three to five hours after your last reasonable eating. That's nothing, right? You can do this! This feeling of hunger registers at around a 3 or 4 on a Hunger Rating Scale of 1 to 10.

A couple of approaches can be beneficial when it comes to eating with hunger. One option is to simply wake up in the morning and wait until you feel physical hunger before you eat. Continue to tune into your physical sensations around your abdomen, noticing if you hear growling, feel hunger pangs, or feel something acidic-like moving around in your stomach. When you feel sufficient hunger, go ahead and eat, staying mindful of your hunger and fullness cues. Take a break when you feel satisfied and wait until you feel hunger before eating again.

Another approach is to make a plan of approximately what times you will eat (for example, early morning, mid-morning, noon, mid-afternoon, and around dinner time). By doing so, you can go ahead and eat early in the morning before a job that doesn't let you step away to eat when you feel physical hunger (nurses and teachers come to mind). At each predetermined eating time, you can then decide a) whether or not you even feel hunger and b) how much you will actually eat. Sometimes, you will not feel hunger at those times and you may choose to wait to eat until you feel the sensation of hunger. Other times, you will feel hungry at that time. The more you practice waiting for hunger and stopping when you are satisfied, your eating will fall into a predictable rhythm.

It's also helpful to anticipate times of eating when you will want to be hungry (special outings or family suppers, for example). During the eating period just before that meal, anticipate and let that guide how much you eat, so you will feel hunger a few hours later when you are at the group gathering or meal. "Saving your hunger" for those gatherings helps you eat within your hunger/fullness window.

Again, start your eating by asking God to help you eat "just enough" (Proverbs 25:16) and to help you stop when you are satisfied, not stuffed. During my own healing period, I often included this prayer when saying the blessing before my meals: "Thank you for this food. Please help me stop when I've had enough."

Once you choose what you want to eat and begin eating, stay aware. Slowing down your eating helps you pay attention to what you are tasting, deciding if you even like it, asking yourself if you are even hungry for it, then knowing when you're finished. In my house, we used to sing a song to help our young girls with this practice: "Eat slowly, you'll be happy long! Eat quickly, you'll be sad it's gone."

It is also helpful to be fully present with your food (and your friends, family, or coworkers), instead of eating while doing something else like scrolling through social media or watching TV. Not rushing or multitasking while you eat lets you enjoy the experience of eating with hunger—you can actually think about how the food tastes. Is it salty, sweet, crunchy, smooth, cold, hot, warm? Go slowly and enjoy one bite (or peanut M&M!) at a time. Continue to check in with yourself and ask yourself if you are hungry as you eat.

Keep in mind that the food you ate at your last meal or snack will impact how much hunger you feel at the current meal. It's also rare for the amount of food on your plate to be an exact match for the amount of hunger in your body. Why would it be? Knowing this, you can begin to eat, knowing that you will either have more food than you're hungry for in front of you or less than you're hungry for. I once backpacked through Europe and a friend advised me to lay out everything I thought I'd need, then take half of it because I probably was packing too much. This approach has helped me with food as well. I like to start with half of what I think I'll need, then add more if I'm still hungry when I finish.

Be selective about which foods you put on your plate. When choosing food, I tell myself, "Love it or leave it," because I do not want to waste stomach space on food that I don't even like or is of mediocre quality. For example, I love milk chocolate, so when it comes to Halloween candy, I don't give a second glance to Nerds or Jolly Ranchers because they contain zero chocolate. When you start with the foods you like the most, it will be easier to stop eating when you're satisfied because you've already eaten the foods you really like. You aren't missing out because you already enjoyed your favorites.

A plan is also helpful. Just as you would not visit a new city without thinking about the highlights and tourist attractions you'd like to see, you'll make the most of your day if you have an idea of what you want to eat. Certain foods, like fruits, vegetables, and whole grains, offer nutrition and other benefits. Meeting with a nutritionist, even once, is a great way to learn about which foods benefit your body. Many employers' health insurance providers offer free health coaching services to help you learn ways to care for your health through meal planning and food preparation. Before going to work, plan ahead and pack your lunch with specific foods you'll want to eat later, so that you're not stuck staring at a snack machine choosing between two kinds of undesirable, processed potato chips. When I hadn't made a plan for the day, I sometimes ended up buying something comparable to "gas station food" (as I like to call it) out of a snack machine only because that was the food available to me in the building where I worked. With your freedom, think ahead and pack beneficial and appealing foods for later in the day.

Planning also helps you be practical about how much you eat and when. Some jobs don't permit you to step away and eat at the exact moment you feel physical hunger. It's helpful to anticipate those circumstances. I've encouraged teachers to wake up and eat something that will give them sustained energy for their morning, but then attentively wait for hunger once they have more power over how they spend their day. In the same way, if you'd like to feel hunger when your family gathers for an evening meal or when you plan to meet a friend for dinner, let that guide how much you eat when you feel hungry for your afternoon snack so you can feel hunger a few hours later. Planning helps us balance our hunger cues with what is practical.

As you follow your hunger cues, you'll start to notice things in our culture and in the environment around you that tempt you to eat without hunger. Candy bars were recently placed near the return desk of a popular store in town; it hadn't even occurred to me to eat chocolate when I just needed to return a set of lightbulbs, but now it does! The size of plates has also increased dramatically since the 1950s when people didn't seem to struggle with overeating. Portion sizes at restaurants are enough for two to three meals when you really focus on how much your body is physically hungry for.

Speaking of portions, I've found it helpful to buy single portions of foods that I'd like to enjoy but not binge on. You can find single portions of kettle chips, ice cream, and other "treats." Don't worry if it isn't cost-efficient to buy a single serving. You might save money in the long run on medical bills by enjoying a single portion at a time.

During the Releasity course, we practice slow, mindful eating with either a strawberry or a grape. I give participants the instructions for eating in a "No-FFFLY" zone. This is a helpful acronym that assists us with slowing our pace to appreciate our food and recognize when we are filling up:

- NON-dominant hand (eat with the hand you don't usually use)

- One bite at a time

- Fork down between bites

- Focus on your food—How does it taste? What is its temperature and texture?

- Finish what's in your mouth before you take another bite

- Look around you (enjoy the people and places you can see)

- Yahweh (ask God for help)

HOW TO STOP WHEN YOU ARE SATISFIED

Keep praying! Ask God to help you stop when you've had "just enough." Trust me, He has so many more interesting things for you to do in life than overeat. He made you to love people, experience His creation, be creative, and bring order to your home and community. He's glad for you to take a break from eating and He will help you find something else to do! I promise you will feel hunger again soon and will enjoy more food later. Remember that you will likely feel hunger three to five hours after you last ate if you stopped when you were physically satisfied.

Stay aware as you eat to recognize what I like to call the "Lord's Last Call." A bartender lets people know it's closing time by shouting, "Last call!" Similarly, your stomach sends a subtle message to your brain that says, "We are starting to fill up. You probably should stop eating in the next few bites." You might rate your fullness/hunger on the scale when you have a feeling that it's time to slow down. Even though this moment isn't always terribly fun for me (especially when I'm eating Indian food or kettle chips), I do feel good when I have moved on to my next activity and can avoid the discomfort of an overstuffed stomach. You will find something else to do with your time and can enjoy your leftovers later. Trust your stomach and trust God. When it comes to food, it may not always feel good to stop, but it always feels good to not be stuffed.

SOCIAL SITUATIONS

Sometimes you will be in social situations where you don't feel like you have as much power to stop eating or other options of how to spend your time. Here are a few tips for those moments.

At a restaurant, ask your server what the most popular menu items are so you can order the best foods and ones you'll probably enjoy. Look around at the décor or dive into conversation with your tablemate. This may sound crazy, but did you know that you can use your freedom to ask the waiter to not bring the complimentary chips or bread that often arrive at the beginning of the meal, so you'll still have hunger when your menu selection arrives at the table? Plan to enjoy the meal twice and ask your server to go ahead and bring a "to go" box at the beginning of the meal. Cut your burger in half before you start eating because you may not be hungry for the second half of it. The next day, you will be so happy (and your coworkers will be jealous!) when you still have a restaurant meal to enjoy in the staff breakroom. When you have eaten to satisfaction, move your "trigger foods" (the ones you most want to eat when you aren't hungry) out of plain view. Sabotage them by pouring water or hot sauce on them or ask a friend to keep the food at her spot until you've left the restaurant.

Prioritize fun if you're stuck in a meeting with a lot of food on hand. Pretend to take notes but do something more interesting on your notepad, or get engaged in a good conversation with someone sitting next to you. Whatever it takes, find a way to occupy yourself other than by eating. If you're at a gathering, a perfect way to shift away from focusing on the food is to start helping with the clean-up or taking pictures for people. Remind yourself that you are free to stop eating. Remind yourself that God will help you. Remind yourself that you can eat again in three to five hours if you feel hungry and want to.

Have you ever eaten with the world's slowest eaters? My mom practically takes a lifetime to finish a meal. Once, when I was in college and back home for a weekend, I decided to see if I could eat at her pace. She has always maintained a healthy weight (seemingly without trying) and I thought I could learn from her pacing. If she took a bite, I took a bite. If she twirled her glass before drinking out of it, I twirled my glass. Oddly, I learned that my mom has a relaxed way of "raking" her rice with her fork, then smoothing over the top before she puts enough food on her fork to bring it to her mouth. Have fun the next time you're with those "skinny eaters" and "match them." Make it a game and have fun learning.

Some people can be a bad influence when it comes to eating habits, even your closest friends and family. Have your response ready when people pressure you to eat food you don't want. Find a helpful friend at a party who will pray for you; let them know when you're having a hard time and ask them to pray. A friend once pulled me aside at a party and asked me to pray for her because she wasn't connecting with anyone at the party. However, she said, she sure could connect with the "Big B" and pointed to a plate of brownies on the buffet table!

Here's a secret. Sometimes all these ideas just don't work. Sometimes you can't seem to stop eating, but a small part of you still knows it's time to stop. The advice given to me for these moments is to "ask that part of you to pray for you." Find your prayer cheerleaders and get them to commit to praying for you in this. I promise, God will continue to help you and keep moving you forward if you keep seeking His help and giving it your best try; you don't need to do this perfectly.

YOU'VE GOT THIS!

Remember that God gave us internal hunger and fullness cues as a guide and as a gift. The more we tune into them, the closer we grow to God because we come to Him in prayer instead of going to food when we weren't even hungry in the first place. He then meets us and transforms us. We also can become self-aware in other areas of our lives. As we learn to keep out the negative effects of excess food, we begin to recognize other places where we have let in negative influences. This could be the beginning of creating healthy boundaries with our time, our work habits, and our relationships. As we learn to trust our inner voice, we are no longer bound to external voices that make us eat a certain way or negatively influence our lives.

This will be a significant and new *learning process* for you. You are forming new neural pathways and it will not always go perfectly. Some days will be better than others. At first, you'll not eat the way you had hoped and then, only later, you'll remember how you had wanted to eat. But, as you continue to practice, you'll eventually be mindful of how you want to eat *while* you are eating. This moment of awareness will occur earlier and earlier in the process as you learn from your mistakes and try again with the next "waiting for hunger." Eventually, you'll remember *how* you want to eat *before* you eat. This takes practice.

When you eat more than you are physically hungry for, remember to "be curious and not critical" of yourself. Ask yourself why you overate rather than saying unkind things to yourself in your head and out loud. If you are kind to yourself through the mess-ups, rather than being hard on yourself, you can move forward more quickly instead of slowing down your progress because you have to recover from self-condemnation. As you learn to wait for hunger, you will go to God and grow closer to Him than ever before. He isn't mad at you for overeating. He only wants you to come to Him.

SET FREE & SATISFIED

REFLECTION QUESTIONS

Jot down the key ideas covered in this chapter.

Describe your personal history of waiting for hunger before eating. What are examples of times you intentionally waited for hunger before eating or times that you remember feeling hungry?

What were the practices of your family in terms of waiting for hunger or eating according to the clock? What are some reasons that your family did or did not eat according to hunger and fullness cues?

What are some examples from your life of ignoring your hunger and fullness cues in order to follow diets or other man-made food rules?

EAT WITH HUNGER WHEN YOU FEEL IT

What are your thoughts toward waiting for hunger to eat and stopping when you feel satisfied? In what ways are these thoughts negative or positive?

_____

_____

_____

_____

JOURNALING

Set a timer for five minutes and write any thoughts or reflections you have. Write down any recent challenges or victories you have experienced related to your body, eating, or your emotions. Use the space below to write during the five minutes.

_____

_____

_____

_____

_____

_____

MEMORIZE

Choose one of the following verses and write it on an index card or Post-it Note where you can see it each day. Try to say it out loud daily and commit it to memory during this week.

"I am the LORD your God, who brought you up out of Egypt. Open wide your mouth and I will fill it."
—Psalm 81:10

"If you find honey, eat just enough—too much of it, and you will vomit."
—Proverbs 25:16

Copy this verse in the space below as you begin to commit it to memory. If you choose a different verse, write it in the space below.

_____

_____

_____

_____

PRAYER

Check in with your friend who is supporting you in prayer. This is a perfect week to ask for prayer that you will learn how to follow your internal hunger and fullness cues for eating. Take a moment to write your own prayer to God in the space below.

_____

_____

_____

_____

_____

PRACTICE

Remember to show yourself love and self-care.

Spend this week trying to wait for hunger before you eat. Be sure to ask God to help you! Choose one of two approaches for this:

- Free-form—Wake up in the morning and wait until you feel physically hungry before you eat. Be sure to ask God to help you wait for hunger and stop when you are satisfied. Be careful not to go more than five hours between eating.

- Plan—Decide in advance what times you'd like to eat (for example, early morning, mid-morning, lunchtime, afternoon snack, dinner) and identify some choice foods you'd like to have on hand. At those designated times, ask

God to help you eat if you are hungry and help you eat as much as you are physically hungry for.

Spend some time searching online for a hunger/fullness scale that you like. Save a screenshot of the scale or print it to help you gauge your hunger and fullness cues as you go about your day.

Keep a list of the "alternate activities" you find to do while you wait for hunger. You can share these with a friend who struggles with overeating, or save them as ideas of what you can do in the future when you wait for hunger.

CHAPTER 6

Acknowledge Your Emotions

The heart has its reasons of which reason knows nothing.
—Blaise Pascal

August 2021 was a rough month for my family. It started when I had an accident while walking down a hill. Yes, just by simply walking downhill. I tripped on my uneven street, tumbled to the pavement, and rolled a few more feet. When all was said and done, I had scraped both palms, knees, and a touch of my legs.

Only a few days later, my daughter had an accident at our community pool when she tried to exit the pool too fast and fell face forward onto the pavement, leading to a laceration in her eyelid and a trip to the emergency room. In both cases, we needed medical attention by way of bandages, antibiotics, and even some expensive

$2,000 medical glue to put my daughter's eyelid back together. Thankfully, we got what we needed and began to heal.

But imagine if we hadn't gotten medical attention. Imagine if I'd tumbled down that hill and a neighbor had offered to help with an ice cream cone and some chocolate cake. What if a lifeguard had brought my child a banana split instead of a bandage for her split eyelid? You'd think this was ridiculous, and so would I. In those cases, we wouldn't take our physical pain to food. Somehow, though, many people have gotten in the habit of taking emotional pain to food for some relief.

We are now at Step 5 of Releasity: **Acknowledge Your Emotions. This is also the second piece of the daily rhythm acronym, HELP: to name your "emotions" when you want to eat but aren't physically hungry.** 1 Corinthians 6:13 says, "Food for the stomach and the stomach for food." As you've taken a week to practice eating when you feel physical hunger, you probably realize you've been using the food for far more than the stomach's original design and intention. We often use food to avoid unpleasant emotions or to be our companion as we feel unpleasant emotions. We eat more than we are physically hungry for as a way of celebrating our happy emotions, or we eat to celebrate being away from something unhappy. In short, we just eat *with our emotions.* Instead of eating only when we feel hunger in our stomachs, we eat when we feel uncomfortable in our hearts. In order to reach our healthy, ideal weight, we need to return to an appropriate practice of using food to fill our stomachs, not our hearts as a way of dealing with our emotions.

In this chapter, we will explore just what our hearts were made for and how we can appropriately care for them, rather than eating when we have unrest in them. We've been taking our emotions to food and not to God—we want to change that path today and begin

ACKNOWLEDGE YOUR EMOTIONS

taking our emotions to God and letting Him help us handle them in a healthy way.

First, it's important to know that **God gave us our hearts and our emotions, even the unpleasant ones.** While some people want to believe that emotions are simply an evolutionary trait we have for survival (and fear does help us run from bears and survive), the Bible teaches that we are made in God's image. God didn't need emotions to survive so that can't be the whole story. Rather, we share in God's display of emotions when we experience them. Many Scripture passages reference God's emotions. Jesus wept (John 11:35) and felt anger (Mark 3:5). God felt compassion (Psalm 119:77) and joy (Zephaniah 3:17). If we know God felt and feels emotions and we are made in His image *with emotions*, we must ask why we have them. I believe emotions show us the significance of moments and add colors to the figurative canvas of our lives, helping our brains and hearts process, identify, and express what's going on.

Emotions help us appreciate good things like beautiful sunsets, generous gifts, a wonderful relationship, or an adorable baby or child. Emotions also raise our awareness when aspects of life aren't good, fair, or healthy, so that we can do something about it. Emotions help motivate us to change. They help us see that things are bad and that we can grieve the loss of the good. I once heard at a funeral that "grief is the evidence of love." In *Shadowlands*, a film about author C. S. Lewis's life, we watch his character struggle through his dying wife's last days. As they reflect on the good times they enjoyed earlier in their relationship, she reminds him, "The pain now is part of the happiness then. That's the deal."[1] All emotions have a purpose.

As for the heart, in addition to being a physical organ that pumps blood, we also refer to our "heart" as the place where our emotions are felt. We know that God has a heart because of verses like 1 Samuel

13:14, which says, "The Lord has sought for Himself a man after His own heart." Our hearts are also an example of how we are made in His image. So, just what were God's intentions when He gave us these hearts with all the feelings they contain?

First, the Bible says we are meant to connect with God and other people through our hearts. In Luke 10:27, Jesus was recorded as saying, "Love the Lord your God with all your heart and with all your soul and with all your strength and with all your mind," and "Love your neighbor as yourself." God hopes for us to be in relationship with Him and other humans through the ways we use our hearts and express and experience our feelings. Paul wrote in Philippians 1:4 and 1:7, "In all my prayers for all of you, I always pray with joy because of your partnership in the gospel. . . . It is right for me to feel this way about all of you, since I have you in my heart." God gave us hearts to have "all the feels," as they say, and to communicate those "feels."

God also gave us hearts so we could know Him better. Jeremiah 24:7 says, "I will give them a heart to know me, that I am the LORD. They will be my people, and I will be their God, for they will return to me with all their heart." "To know God with our hearts" refers to relational connection, not simply "knowing of" God like someone we've never met. As for God, having you return to Him with *all* of your heart matters to him! God invites you to come to Him with everything you are feeling—your joys, sorrows, fears, confusion, doubts, hopes, and dreams. You can bring it all to Him. Jesus said, "Come to me, all you who are weary and burdened, and I will give you rest" (Matthew 11:28).

The problem is we don't always know how to handle our emotions properly, and we've used food to numb or avoid our feelings for so long. It's true that we don't want our emotions to overtake us, but we've erred in completely avoiding them and running to food.

Sometimes we go to food to "help our hearts" because we don't know how to cope with the specific issue that's leading us to overeat, but we are well accustomed to being upset about our overeating.

However, for some of us, another factor is at play. Research has shown that 30 percent of adults with binge-eating disorder (consuming large amounts of calories at one sitting and feeling intense regret afterward) also have a history of Attention Deficit Hyperactivity Disorder (ADHD).[2] One of the characteristics of ADHD is a difficulty with effectively regulating emotions. Further research has shown that people with ADHD register a higher "reward" in the brain when presented with food than a person who does not have characteristics of ADHD.[3] This all adds up to a concerning combination of risks when it comes to emotions, food, and our brains.

Sometimes, we learn to take our emotions to food by watching others overeat, or we learn it through trial and error. We may have started going to food for emotional reasons as a kid or as an adult. Do you remember when this habit started for you?

We isolate ourselves from people and God and eat rather than directly deal with what's bothering us. It's less demanding, but we miss out on deep, authentic intimacy with God and people. This is our loss. In the book *Addiction and Grace,* author Gerald May noted how "'Saint Augustine once said that God is always trying to give good things to us, but our hands are too full to receive them.' If our hands are full, they are full of the things to which we are addicted. And not only our hands, but also our hearts, minds and attention are clogged with addiction. Our addictions fill up the spaces within us, spaces where grace might flow."[4]

In the case of our painful or unpleasant emotions, when we go to food rather than going to God, we miss out on God's comforting touch to address our pain. In a counseling session, Patti once asked me, "What would happen if you stayed in your room and cried when you're sad, rather than going to the kitchen to eat about it?"

I wanted to quip, "What would happen if I stopped coming to you, lady?" but I refrained. She was right in naming that I was avoiding my feelings by eating.

GOD HAS A BETTER PLAN FOR US

Thankfully, there's more to the story. God has a better, healthier, more life-giving plan for how to deal with our unpleasant or uncomfortable emotions and eat in a reasonable way. By overeating to avoid emotions, we have numbed our hearts into a state of callousness. God wants to transform our hearts and help us feel again and directly cope with our difficult emotions in a constructive way that doesn't involve food as a healing agent. He never meant for us to desensitize ourselves in such a way that we are unable to feel the highs and lows of life. Wouldn't you love to live your life not running to food every time you felt unsettled? I can attest that God brought this transformation in my own life, even when I didn't realize this was my tendency in the first place. He is faithful! God wants to help us handle our emotions so they don't dominate us and lead us to self-destructive behaviors like overeating. He wants us to experience true joy and intimacy with Him and with others. In doing so, we develop understanding and are healed.

How will He do this? It will be like heart surgery. More specifically, it will be a heart transplant. Ezekiel 36:26 says, "I will give you a new heart and put a new spirit in you; I will remove from you your heart of stone and give you a heart of flesh." If this sounds like an unpleasant procedure, I can't lie. It's not always easy. Still, eventually, you will love your new way of operating. It will take courage, but the outcome is a transformed life. You won't eat to deal with your problems, you'll have a more intimate relationship with God and people, and you'll appreciate more of what God intended for you to appreciate in life—beyond chocolate and waffle fries. You will begin to recognize the areas of dysfunction in your life and take steps toward healthy change.

How does this new heart work? In Matthew 13:14–15, Jesus quoted the prophet Isaiah: "You will be ever hearing but never understanding; you will be ever seeing but never perceiving. For this people's heart has become calloused; they hardly hear with their ears, and they have closed their eyes. Otherwise they might see with their eyes, hear with their ears, understand with their hearts and turn, and I would heal them." God's goal is for us to "understand with our hearts." He wants us to bring our emotions (and the situations that cause them) to Him so that we can directly cope with them and experience His love and help, rather than gain weight over our problems that had nothing to do with food in the first place!

God wants to transform our minds and open the eyes of our hearts so we can be aware of the fullness of life He gives, including emotions that range from pure joy to grief at the loss of something that has been profoundly special to us. Paul wrote to the church members of Ephesus:

> I pray that the eyes of your heart may be enlightened
> in order to know the hope to which he has called you,
> the riches of his glorious inheritance in his holy people,
> and his incomparably great power for us who believe.
> That power is the same as the mighty strength he exerted
> when he raised Christ from the dead and seated him at
> his right hand in the heavenly realms, far above all rule
> and authority, power and dominion, and every name

that is invoked, not only in the present age but also in the one to come. And God placed all things under his feet and appointed him to be head over everything for the church, which is his body, the fullness of him who fills everything in every way. (Ephesians 1:18–23)

In Paul's words, you'll see that the goal is for us to be enlightened and have understanding in our hearts—rather than numbing our emotions—to know the hope God has called us to, to understand the wonderful inheritance we have waiting for us, and to recognize God's power to help those of us who believe in Him. Food and/or being thin is no longer the authority in our lives—Jesus is. He even says He will "fill everything in every way"! That speaks to my hungry heart. How about you? Understanding leads to hope, hope leads to focusing on our inheritance, and our inheritance reminds us of our power and that we will be filled in every way. We won't need food to fill our hearts anymore.

The above passage from Ephesians reminds us that God has the power to change any situation and He wants you to be hopeful. He is saying, "Open your eyes and *have hope* because all power is mine!" If we come to him with our emotions and our heart, He will help us with whatever is causing these uncomfortable and painful emotions. He will meet us in our pain and provide comfort rather than leaving us to feel like orphans who have no one to care for them and who must use food to avoid problems. The questions you must ask yourself are, "Can I trust God?" and "Can I wait on Him to work things out for my good?"

As God helps us grow in the spiritual fruit of patience, we will experience the truth of God's promise in Romans 8:28: "And we know that in all things God works for the good of those who love him, who have been called according to his purpose." We no longer let emotions wreck us, nor do we avoid them. We bring them to God and let Him

DIGGING DEEPER

Some of you will need help naming your emotions as you get started. I've been there. Shortly after I learned how to wait for physical hunger, I was at a missionary training where they offered free counseling sessions for a couple of weeks. I'd never met Sandy, the counselor, but I told her about the food healing journey I was on. After a bit, she asked if I knew what I was feeling when I wanted to eat but didn't feel physically hungry.

I leaned in and seriously asked her, "No, do you?"

She contained her amusement at the fact that I imagined she, a stranger, might know what I was thinking or feeling. As she stood up, she said, "Let's take a walk." Sandy ushered me to the children's section of the building. I remember walking past the children playing with each other and thinking, *I wonder what she has for me that is designed for children, yet she thinks I need it as an adult.*

Sandy gave me a chart with a variety of emotions pictured on it. Its heading read, "How Are You Feeling Today?" Sandy told me to keep this sheet of paper close by, and when I wanted to eat but did not feel physically hungry, to look at this sheet and name what I was feeling. This moment was revolutionary for me; I had never been asked to name my emotions.

The very next day while at a shopping mall, I heard the song "Stronger" by Britney Spears. When Britney proclaimed in the end of the chorus that loneliness wasn't killing her anymore, I knew those words oddly described the new path I was taking with my emotions. Acknowledging them and handling them in a healthy way would set me free from eating excess food. God was doing the heart transplant in my life, taking me from being calloused with my emotions to being enlightened. I was starting to realize that overeating because of unpleasant emotions only made everything worse.

You do have a role and a responsibility in all of this. How do you go in for heart surgery and access this transformation God wants to create in your life? First, continue following your internal hunger and fullness cues you learned in Step 4: Eat with Hunger When You Feel It. Pay attention to your stomach and make sure you feel hunger or hear hunger rumblings before you eat.

Second, when you want to eat but aren't physically hungry, ask God to help you identify what you are feeling. In the back of this book, you'll find an "Emotions Wheel" that will help you describe your feelings in the moments when you want to eat but don't feel hunger. Visit the Releasity website for a color PDF of this chart.

Third, when you try to name what you are feeling rather than automatically eating, the best step you can take is to either get rid of the food that is tempting you or physically move away from it. Going to another room or taking a walk outside in the fresh air has often helped me in these moments. Take five minutes alone, outside your house, so you can quietly talk to God and see His imprint in nature.

After you are still and at a safe distance from the food, you can decide what to do next. It's beneficial to invite God into the problem. Pray and tell Him what you are feeling when you want to eat but aren't hungry. It's also helpful to text a friend and ask for prayer in that moment. When you invite a friend into it, the enemy of your soul is no longer keeping you in isolation, and your healing can take place. If you hand over this difficulty to God, He will not leave you empty-handed or carelessly tell you to figure it out on your own. He promises to give you what you need in your trouble. Let Jesus

ACKNOWLEDGE YOUR EMOTIONS

comfort you. Tell Him, for example, "Jesus, I am lonely. Will you please keep me company?"

Finally, after you've been still and shared your emotions with God through prayer, ask the Holy Spirit to guide you. Remember Isaiah 30:21: "Whether you turn to the right or to the left, your ears will hear a voice behind you, saying, 'This is the way; walk in it.'" God wants to guide you through the leading of the Holy Spirit. A few options of how you can respond are listed below:

- Deal with the actual problem if you have the power to do so. Proverbs 3:27 says, "Do not withhold good from those to whom it is due, when it is in your power to act." You may not have full control, but you do have some power to bring about change with God's help.

- Choose to invite others in and call a friend for relational connection.

- Do something nice for someone else. We can take our minds off ourselves and be blessed just by serving someone else. Proverbs 11:25 says, "Whoever refreshes others will be refreshed."

- Take this time for some alone time and self-care, relaxing and refreshing yourself. Trim your nails, take a walk, or rest on your bed or couch. Self-care may also mean using your voice to contend with others when you've been mistreated. While the Bible says "it is to one's glory to overlook an offense" (Proverbs 19:11), it is also helpful sometimes to tell someone when their words or actions have hurt you. At times, you must give your relationships the honesty they deserve and have an open conversation to speak up for yourself. Instead of letting a hurtful comment come into your heart and cause you to overeat, you can say to the person who spoke it, "It hurt my feelings when you said _____."

- The Holy Spirit may lead you to be productive with your time as you practice self-care. Does a load of laundry need to be returned to its drawers? Does a bill need to be paid? Maybe you've been procrastinating with the next step in a situation, and this time of waiting for the next hunger cue is a perfect time to take action.

- Because eating is a sensory experience, you may find comfort in seeking some other kind of sensory input when you want to eat but don't feel hungry. In these moments, I sneak away to take a bath just to feel the warmth of the bath water. Try lighting a candle to enjoy the smell of peppermint on a cold evening. Are there any sensory experiences you enjoy that might offer a reprieve while you wait for the next round of hunger cues? Thankfully, hunger will come again, and you'll enjoy eating knowing you didn't keep eating through your satiated and overly emotional state.

A QUICK WARNING LABEL

Just like a TV commercial for a drug, you should be warned that this new approach to handling emotions comes with potential side effects. Acknowledging your emotions will take time and practice, just like learning how to ride a bicycle. If the practice of sitting with your emotions is new to you, you may have some bumpy spots, like the following:

ACKNOWLEDGE YOUR EMOTIONS

1. It may feel uncomfortable and unfamiliar for a time to not participate in the old, familiar "sad to eat" cycle. This doesn't mean it's wrong. The chain smoker who decides to quit smoking also feels discomfort on the first morning without a cigarette, but that doesn't mean he's doing something wrong. You are not doing something wrong by dodging the kitchen the next time you feel sad but aren't physically hungry.

2. You may cry a lot at first. If you have been numbing your emotions for a long time, you may start to feel sadness that has been buried for years. Many tears may come, but you will survive. If you find that you cannot function to perform your daily responsibilities, you may want to talk with a doctor or counselor about appropriate next steps and the possible use of medication to help with the transition.

3. You may verbally explode on unassuming people. For years, if someone bothered me, I would eat rather than address it with them. Once I stopped the "sad to eat" cycle, I began to speak up for myself, and it wasn't always pretty. If you do not speak the truth in love, you may want to have a follow-up conversation to make peace with the one you hurt.

4. You might unknowingly shift your addictive tendency to someone or something other than food if you don't see God as the one who will ultimately satisfy you. Start by being still with God rather than immediately calling a person to take the place of the food. Humans will always disappoint you in some way, and you want to avoid

125

unhealthy, toxic relationships. Seek God, because He will satisfy you in a way that people simply cannot. Run to God, not another addiction or codependent relationship as you learn to stop going to food to cope.

By "acknowledging our emotions" and taking the uncomfortable ones to God, we begin to break the cycle of "I feel sad, I'm going to eat." Instead, the pattern becomes, "I feel sad, I'm going to talk to God. He will help me process this emotion and problem and lead me to something else."

The more you practice this, along with being kind to yourself because "kinder is faster," being "curious, not critical," and remembering this is "Holy Spirit help, not self-help," you will develop new lifetime habits and keep off the excess weight. You are transforming your mind and being renewed. You are literally forming new neural pathways as you choose healthier routes out of sadness rather than harming your body. Remember Romans 12:2, which says, "Do not conform to the pattern of this world, but be transformed by the renewing of your mind. Then you will be able to test and approve what God's will is—his good, pleasing, and perfect will."

In the past, when something upset me or made me nervous, my gut reaction was to go to the kitchen. Now, by God's grace, on a good day, I think, *I'm upset but I am not going to gain weight over this problem. This problem has nothing to do with food.* God has helped me take my problems to Him more and more in prayer.

As we receive the love, tenderness, and care of Jesus, we learn how to love ourselves and value ourselves. Miraculously and eventually, we no longer want to harm our bodies by overeating. We begin to treat ourselves well and make wise choices to care for ourselves. We begin to eat and live in healthy ways. We have a new heart and a new mind, and our behavior with food follows. We are transformed.

ACKNOWLEDGE YOUR EMOTIONS

REFLECTION QUESTIONS

Jot down the key ideas covered in this chapter.

_____

_____

_____

_____

What are some ways that you feel comfortable or uncomfortable acknowledging your emotions? What are examples of times that you may have been told that your emotions were wrong or that you shouldn't give them merit?

_____

_____

_____

_____

When looking back on your journey with overeating, can you identify a time or times in your life when you began overeating to cope with what you were feeling in your heart? Describe some of those times below.

_____

_____

_____

_____

What scenarios come to mind when you think about being still with your uncomfortable emotions rather than numbing your emotions with food? Describe how this makes you feel, whether excitement or dread.

_____

_____

_____

_____

What are some other sensory experiences you might enjoy rather than going to food when you feel uncomfortable or upset?

_____

_____

_____

_____

What are some positive ways you can care for your heart rather than eating to "cope" with your emotions?

_____

_____

_____

_____

ACKNOWLEDGE YOUR EMOTIONS

JOURNALING

Set a timer for five minutes and write any thoughts or reflections you have after reading this chapter. Use the space below to write during the five minutes.

SET FREE & SATISFIED

MEMORIZE

Write the following verse (or another of your choice) on an index card or Post-it Note where you can see it each day. Try to say it out loud daily and commit it to memory during this week.

"I will give them a heart to know me, that I am the LORD. They will be my people, and I will be their God, for they will return to me with all their heart."
—Jeremiah 24:7

Copy this verse in the space below as you begin to commit it to memory. If you choose a different verse, write it in the space below.

_____

_____

_____

_____

_____

PRAYER

Take a few minutes to write a prayer to the Lord, telling Him or asking Him why you eat when you aren't physically hungry. Ask Him to give you His promises and tell you how He wants to care for you and provide for you in your present difficulty. After you have written, draw two horizontal lines under your prayer, then wait silently. Write down any words, pictures, or Scriptures that come to you, taking time to let the Lord speak to you during your prayer time.

ACKNOWLEDGE YOUR EMOTIONS

PRACTICE

Remember to show yourself love and self-care.

Begin using the Emotions Wheel this week. When you aren't hungry but want to eat, ask God to help you identify what you are feeling.

Take your emotions to God throughout the day through ongoing prayer. You can pour these out to Him in complete honesty. Consider seeing a Christian counselor to learn how to identify and deal with your emotions in a healthy way.

CHAPTER 7

Seek the Spirit Every Day

*So I say, walk by the Spirit, and you will not
gratify the desires of the flesh.*
—Galatians 5:16

As a teenager, I was absolutely boy crazy. At any moment, on any day, I was usually in love with someone. It didn't matter if the object of my affection didn't reciprocate; I resolutely maintained my love for them until I found a new person to fall in love with. My heart's affection steadily bumped along from boy to boy.

My love for food has operated similarly. As I began to recognize the lie of believing that food could solve my problems, I began to lose my love for food. I started to understand that I was made to wait for physical hunger before eating and find something else to do with my time until I felt hunger again. When this happened, I realized there was an affection in my heart that needed a new place to go. If I wasn't going to be in love with food any longer, what could I be in love with? In the same way I kept thinking about a former crush until a new crush came along, my heart's affection for food had to find a new object for its love.

As I mentioned in the risks section of Acknowledge Your Emotions, we must be careful when we stop overeating to not transfer our affection (or addiction) to a new substance or person. If we are ever to find peace with food and not become addicted to a new substance or continuously form bad habits, we must be intentional about learning how to shift our affection away from food to its rightful recipient, the Lord. As Saint Augustine said, "You have made us and drawn us to yourself, and our heart is restless until it rests in you."

While it can be challenging to direct our affections to an invisible God, thankfully He has a plan for how we can connect with Him. After Jesus died on the cross and rose from the dead, ultimately appearing to over five hundred people, the disciples learned He was going away but would send someone else to keep them company. Jesus tells them in John 16:7 and 16:12,

> But very truly I tell you, it is for your good that I am going away. Unless I go away, the Advocate will not come to you; but if I go, I will send him to you. . . . I have much more to say to you, more than you can now bear. But when he, the Spirit of truth, comes, he will guide you into all the truth. He will not speak on his own; he will speak only what he hears, and he will tell you what is yet to come. He will glorify me because it is

from me that he will receive what he will make known to you.

God's design is to be present with us through the Holy Spirit. Learning to draw close to the Spirit, we will redirect our former affection for food to God, its rightful recipient. We are now in the end stretch of the Releasity process at Step Six: **Seek the Spirit Every Day. This is the "L" in our daily rhythm acronym, HELP: Lord.** After we have waited for hunger and named our emotions when we want to eat without hunger, we take those emotions to the Lord.

When we acknowledge our sin and ask Jesus to be our Savior and Lord, God spends time in our presence through the person of the Holy Spirit, a mysterious member of the Trinity (Father, Son, and Holy Spirit). Jesus is unique in that He moves among His people. He is not like the mythical Greek gods or some foreign, false god who doesn't interact with humanity. God is not external to us. He dwells *in us!* All this time, we've been stuffing ourselves with food when God wants to stuff us with His Spirit. When we understand that He dwells in us, that can change us and give us power. To overcome our food addiction, we must enter this new relationship and learn how to show affection and receive the love of God through the Spirit.

When I mention the Holy Spirit, what is your reaction? Are you comfortable, uncomfortable, or neutral? On the one hand, some Christians take the Bible literally when it refers to the Spirit as a "deposit" guaranteeing that Jesus is coming back, and they think of the Spirit as something hidden away like a "deposit" in the bank—as in, *It's mine, but it's locked up at the bank, so I can't easily access it.* When we perceive the Spirit this way, there's little to no interaction occurring.

Other Christians are simply uncomfortable talking about the Holy Spirit. This may be because there have been instances of abuse within some churches that prioritize a focus on the Spirit. Or the term "Holy Ghost" may be scary because we don't typically like to associate with ghosts. Because the Spirit is amorphous, not having a clear shape or form in our understanding, many believers can also feel confused when it comes to interacting with God through His Spirit.

Those mindsets are not beneficial. Jesus said the Holy Spirit would speak to us, and we can trust the Bible's words that the Holy Spirit is here to lovingly communicate God's messages to us. We must seek the Holy Spirit if we are going to be transformed to lose our love for excess food. To learn how to seek the Spirit, let's answer three questions: why, when, and how.

UNDERSTANDING THE SPIRIT

First and foremost, we must seek the Spirit simply because **our very lives depend on it**. In our flesh, we want to eat too much and we go to food as a god. Exodus 22:20 says, "Whoever sacrifices to any god other than the LORD must be destroyed." And Galatians 6:8 tells us, "Whoever sows to please their flesh, from the flesh will reap destruction; whoever sows to please the Spirit, from the Spirit will reap eternal life."

When we turn the food into a god, our thinness into a god, or ourselves into a god, we face great danger. We must learn to bring our flesh into submission to the Spirit because we aren't on Earth to be controlled by our bodies. In my struggle with food and development of bad habits, I had become addicted to overeating, which is not the "full life" Jesus says He came to give me in John 10:10. The Spirit will help us eat in a way that is life-giving rather than idol-making.

If we have children, choosing life through the Spirit also has implications for our family's future generations. I often think of my own struggle with overeating. For generations before me, I know that my family members wrestled with not eating too much. It's not uncommon for overeating to be passed down from grandparent to parent to child. When we seek the Spirit, though, we can break strongholds for our children and future grandchildren. New eating habits can begin to take form for our children and grandchildren.

Pursuing this new life, rather than sin, allows us to follow the Spirit's promptings and spend time in prayer. Rather than bingeing on food we aren't hungry for, we begin to experience God's goodness, mercy, and care for us. We expose the lie of believing food can be a "savior" and a place where we should run and hide. Our perspective is changed and we begin to be accurate about who God says He is. We receive God's love and begin to believe He finds us valuable. This, in turn, causes us to value ourselves. That leads us to eat differently because we want to care for ourselves, not harm ourselves. The transformation has begun.

I once visited a cemetery during the cold winter months. Because of the graves and the winter dormancy of the trees, my mind perceived this graveyard as black and white. I remember thinking I felt like that graveyard because of my anxiety and addiction to eating too much food. As I later began to seek the Spirit and be transformed into feeling more life again, I remember feeling like I had gone from a black-and-white existence to a colorful life. This happens when we actively seek the Spirit and commune with God in this way.

We must also seek the Spirit to obtain **guidance**. It comes in the form of new insight and wisdom as well as experiencing the Spirit guiding us into very practical and helpful next steps in our struggle with food. At this point in the Releasity process, I imagine you have many questions. Jesus said the Holy Spirit will "guide you into all truth" if you will seek Him. He promised, "I have much more to say to you. . . . But when he, the Spirit of truth, comes, he will guide you into all the truth" (John 16:12–13). Take your questions to Jesus and quietly say in prayer, "What are you trying to show me, Lord?"

When I want to eat but don't feel physically hungry, I often lean on the Lord to find my "way of escape." As we wait for hunger before we eat again, we can have a conversational romance with God through His Spirit. It becomes a joy to talk to God throughout the day and wait for a nudge on when to eat next and what to do in the meantime. God will show up when we seek Him instead of the excess food.

Last, we must seek the Spirit to access the **supernatural power** that will bring lasting transformation in our lives. The same power that raised Jesus from the dead after his death on the cross is available to us! Romans 8:26 says, "In the same way, the Spirit helps us in our weakness. We do not know what we ought to pray for, but the Spirit himself intercedes for us through wordless groans."

You will be amazed how much self-control you'll gain when you earnestly seek the Spirit, intentionally setting aside time to pray and ask for new life, guidance, and self-control. The Spirit brings a unique, supernatural transformation that exceeds anything you will read in this book. Remember, diets and eating rules do not have the power to change desires, but God can change your desires! I know women (myself included) who have been set free from shame and mental preoccupation with what they eat and what they look like because of the power of the Holy Spirit.

HOW TO SEEK THE SPIRIT

When exactly should you seek the Spirit? Simply, seek Him "out of the moment" and "in the moment" of your temptation to overeat. "Out of the moment" I find it helpful to commit my needs to the Lord through prayer first thing in the morning. If you're like me and forget to do this, place a Post-it Note as a reminder over your bathroom sink where you first spend time in the morning. On some mornings, I prayed the Lord's prayer (Matthew 6: 9–13), asking God to "lead me not into temptation but deliver me from the evil one." I've asked that He provide a way of escape (1 Corinthians 10:13). I've even claimed 2 Timothy 1:7 for myself: "For the spirit God gave us does not make us timid, but gives us power, love, and self-discipline." I also ask God to give me wisdom (James 1:5) to responsibly use my freedom with food that day.

"In the moment" means talking to the Lord during the exact times you want to eat but are not physically hungry. Ask for help in identifying your feelings and ask for the vocabulary to describe your emotions. In a moment of wanting to eat but not feeling hungry, I feel victorious to be able to say, "I feel anxious and irritable." I couldn't have identified that about myself twenty years ago. In the moments when you have erred to great proportions and overeaten, remember to be "curious and not critical" and to ask the Spirit, "What are you trying to show me?" Practice the phrase "kinder is faster," because shame doesn't motivate us—kindness does.

How do you seek the Spirit? The answer is a bit complex, but a few words starting with "S" can help you remember. Seek the Spirit through:

- **Silence**

- **Scripture**

- **Saying "sorry"** (confession)

- **Surrendering** to what God says is best for you

The first practice, **silence**, goes best with stillness and solitude when we are healing from our addiction to food. The Bible mentions different occasions when Jesus was intentional about being alone in order to connect with God through prayer. In our day and time, unfortunately, we have to work hard to experience solitude, stillness, and silence. Before smartphones, TV, and radio, one often had the chance to be alone and quiet. Now, we only have it forced on us in the shower and in the dentist's chair (and now my dentist's office has a TV screen to distract me!). Even gas pumps have TV screens to keep you occupied while you fill up your gas. Podcasts fill our ears even if we can find time to be alone.

Amid all this distraction, be careful to leave space to hear the Spirit speak to you. We must be intentional in our pursuit of experiencing solitude with God. The Bible includes multiple instances when Jesus made it a point to be alone in order to meet with God. Mark 1:35 says, "Very early in the morning, while it was still dark, Jesus got up, left the house and went off to a solitary place, where he prayed." If Jesus had to rise early to ensure He had time alone with God, don't we need to do this even more?

When I was single, I used to tell my girlfriends that the easiest way to encourage a man to approach them at a party was to "dump the clump." This meant you shouldn't go to an event and stand in a group talking to your girlfriends. It was too intimidating for a guy to come up and talk to you. However, if my friend walked to the side of the room and looked at a piece of art on the wall by herself, nine times out of ten, a guy she didn't know would have the confidence to start a conversation with her. This worked for me so many times in my dating years that on nights when I forgot the principle, I accidentally attracted men simply by standing alone in a public place! The Spirit is similar—you must be alone to have these interactions through prayer. Matthew 6:6 encourages us, "But when you pray, go into your room, close the door and pray to your Father, who is unseen. Then your Father, who sees what is done in secret, will reward you."

We also encounter the Holy Spirit through **Scripture**. Because we have an enemy who regularly lies to us, we must do what Jesus did when he was tempted by Satan. We must speak the truth of Scripture just as Jesus countered Satan's temptations in the desert (Matthew 4:1–11). Our culture and insensitive people have lied to us over the years. Our minds must marinate in God's truth to be transformed. In the parable of the sower in Matthew 13, we read that some people in the world fall victim to Satan "stealing the word" from them. If Satan tries to steal the word from us, the word must be pretty powerful!

It's helpful to have a location in your home designated for your daily, focused time of reading Scripture. My goal is to read one chapter of the Bible each day and perhaps read the same chapter the following day if I want to give a passage extra time to sink in. I may write down a verse or two from the chapter that resonated with me as a way of helping me meditate on the Scripture. This reinforces the verse in my mind and increases the likelihood it will come to mind later in the day. I may also ask myself, *What does this passage tell me about God's character?* or *What does this passage tell me about how people are?* Lastly, I may ask, *How might this passage impact me to live differently, with God's help, in the future?* You may want to purchase a devotional to read alongside your Bible, but I've found it helpful to keep it simple by reading a passage of the Bible daily and thinking about the words that come directly from God.

It's also important to find a Bible you enjoy. Many people are trying to get through the King James Version their dear Aunt Tabitha gave them as a child. I met a woman who showed up at a Bible study in her twenties with the children's Bible she'd been given as a youth; she didn't know there were Bibles geared more toward adults! I love her story, in particular, because her love for God's word eventually led her to become a Bible teacher. Ask a friend or someone at church to help you find a version you can relate to. I particularly enjoy "Study Bibles" and the "Life Application Bible" because they help you connect passages to your day-to-day experience. You can also "follow the trail" of cross references and read other verses that relate to a chapter you enjoy. Popular, easier-to-read versions include the New International Version (NIV), English Standard Version (ESV), and the New Living Translation (NLT).

Memorizing Scripture is a powerful tool. When we have easy mental access to God's Word, it is so refreshing to have something "playing" in our minds rather than anxious thoughts and negative critiques of ourselves. However, this isn't like memorizing information for a boring science test. Finding a verse that really encourages you will aid in your transformation and help you counteract a lie you have been believing. The Bible talks about being renewed by the transforming of your mind, and memorizing Scripture helps with this. Joshua Choonmin Kang writes, "To lead a life in search of wisdom we must learn Scripture by heart. Scripture contains half a dozen major treasuries of practical and spiritual wisdom. When we store them up in our heart, we deepen our reservoir of wisdom.

When we meditate, we lower our ladle into the clear, cool water and refresh our spirit to hitherto unknown heights."[1]

Choose one verse to memorize and write it on an index-card ring, then put the ring over your kitchen sink and leave it for a week or two. The verse will become familiar as you keep meditating on it. In desperate times, I have also written a verse on a small piece of paper and carried it with me throughout the workday, pulling it out of my pocket to read when I have a moment to myself. This gives me another moment of solitude to connect with the Spirit.

When my daughter was three years old, she happened to memorize the words to an Adele song. Do you think I sat down with her and said, "Okay, let's look at these words and try to commit them to memory?" No, I just kept exposing her to the song, unintentionally, because I personally liked the song so much. After hearing it just a few times, she knew all the words by heart. Think of a song you memorized simply because you kept exposing yourself to it out of enjoyment. This is the goal with meditating on and memorizing Scripture. If you're thinking, *That won't work for me; I'm terrible at memorizing,* pray God would give you a hunger for His word and the ability to memorize it. He will!

We also encounter the Spirit through saying the word **"sorry."** It's true that we were born with the freedom to eat what we want, and we cannot lose God's love. Our righteousness before God is completely based on what Jesus did for us on the cross, not because of what we eat or don't eat, what we weigh, or what we look like. However, there are still times when the way we eat can be considered sinful and require that we apologize or say "sorry" to God. Galatians 5:13 says, "You, my brothers and sisters, were called to be free. But do not use your freedom to indulge the flesh; rather, serve one another humbly in love." I believe that my overeating becomes a sin when it is gluttonous, or when it becomes an idol for me. I'll explain.

Proverbs 23:20–21 says, "Do not join those who drink too much wine or gorge themselves on meat, for drunkards and gluttons become poor, and drowsiness clothes them in rags." The Bible also says to put a knife to your throat "if you are given to gluttony" (Proverbs 23:2). *Ouch.* I don't believe God really wants us to cut our throats, but this verse tells us how seriously we should take a habit of gluttony in our lives.

The bottom line is that we are called by God to care for our bodies. For those of us who have asked Jesus to be our Savior, our body is the temple of the Holy Spirit (1 Corinthians 6:19). Many people have used this verse to motivate people to live a healthy lifestyle, but it can also be the means for a guilt trip. This tactic has yet to work for me because it made me feel bad about myself. Instead, the Bible says God's kindness—not a guilt trip—is what leads us to repentance or change.

With that in mind, let's look at our sin in light of God's kindness. For me, the fact that I have gone to food for comfort and connection—and in the process have made food an idol—is more impactful as I think of why I should repent. God wants my heart while I instead repeatedly give it to food. God is a jealous God. He is jealous when I trust food instead of Him, and this motivates me to change. I want to respond to God's love with love, not by avoiding Him and eating extra food. Another motivation for me to apologize is that I have made an idol, or false god, of my appearance. I realized years ago that I wanted to be pretty and thin more than I wanted to be able to walk! I was worshipping thinness and needed to confess this sin to my loving God. I also idolized the praise of others and would pridefully seek out compliments for my weight loss.

How do you feel when I encourage you to apologize to God or confess your sin? If it makes you uncomfortable, let me encourage you that confession is a good thing. Jesus said, "I tell you that in the same way there will be more rejoicing in heaven over one sinner who repents than over ninety-nine righteous persons who do not need to repent" (Luke 15:7). Did you catch that? There's *rejoicing* in heaven when there is repentance on Earth! Confession is even a celebration that precedes transformation. When we confess, God forgives us and His power to transform us is unleashed. 1 John 1:9 says, "If we confess our sins, he is faithful and just and will forgive us our sins and purify us from all unrighteousness." When we confess overeating and making an idol of food or our appearance, God forgives us and begins to purify us.

This is the simplest explanation of how I've been able to lose almost fifty pounds and keep it off for over twenty years. When I overeat, I tell God I am sorry for turning to the food for comfort or worship, instead of relying on Him. He forgives me and purifies me, bringing lasting, supernatural transformation, causing me to eat just what I need and not binge any longer. With 2 Corinthians 12:9 as my model, I can "boast all the more gladly about my weakness so Christ's power may rest on me." It is a good thing to confess and admit where we are weak; that's when the healing starts. Putting it all together, it's amazing to think of all the positive words we can now associate with saying "sorry" and confessing our sin: kindness (Romans 2:4), rejoicing (Luke 15:7), purification (1 John 1:9), and refreshing (Acts 3:19).

Confession also has a positive impact on our earthly relationships. Dietrich Bonhoeffer, a German pastor who lived in the mid-1900s wrote,

> In confession there takes place a breakthrough to
> community. Sin wants to be alone with people. It takes
> them away from the community. The more lonely people
> become, the more destructive the power of sin over
> them. The more deeply they become entangled in it,
> the more unholy is their loneliness. Sin wants to remain
> unknown. . . . In confession the light of the gospel
> breaks into the darkness and closed isolation of the heart.
> Sin must be brought into the light.[2]

A regular feature of our in-person Releasity groups is a sharing time when participants are invited to speak aloud without interruption. Often, it becomes a healing time where people share their mistakes with food and their regrets. I'm convinced the confession nature of this time helps brings healing.

Finally, we must **surrender our wills** to God. We often think of weight loss as a battle with food and our flesh. However, Ephesians 6:12 says the fight isn't against the flesh but "against the rulers, against the authorities, against the powers of this dark world and against the spiritual forces of evil in the heavenly realms." I've learned it's not as much combat against weight or food as much as a battle about surrendering to God and allowing Him to be victorious for me in the spiritual realm. This sets me free from overeating. The question then becomes, *Whose plan will prevail, mine or God's?* Will God's prescribed boundaries with food ultimately lead to my freedom, or will I insist on my self-satisfying and destructive desires?

The Bible's definition of "obey" is to "submit to the voice that is heard." Many of you are beginning to hear a voice that is saying, "You don't need that extra piece of cake; it can't do for you what you need, but I can." We show God we love Him by obeying this voice (John

14:15). The wonderful outcome is that, when we submit to God, we win as well. As we submit to His pleasant eating boundaries for us, we avoid the shame and guilt of overeating, reach our healthy weight, and possibly avoid weight-related medical problems down the road. We must surrender to God if we are ever going to have peace.

Seeking the Spirit is a lifelong process as we continue learning how to let our affections rest on God rather than food. My prayer is that we will be like the bleeding woman mentioned in Mark 5 who wholeheartedly pursued Jesus to be healed. She believed that, just by getting near Him and touching him, she would be healed, even after years of spending her money on other attempts. Does this multi-year, costly pursuit of health sound familiar? After she secretly touched Him in the crowd, Jesus knew His power had gone out to someone. Once He identified her, Jesus said to her, "Daughter, your faith has healed you. Go in peace and be freed from your suffering" (Mark 5:34).

As you seek the Spirit, you too can be freed from your suffering. It's tempting to try and lose weight by focusing on external food rules and fad diets, but let me remind you that Jesus said you must wash the inside of the cup for the outside to be transformed. Seeking the Spirit is how you wash the inside of the cup. The true, lifelong solution is internal, not external.

SET FREE & SATISFIED

REFLECTION QUESTIONS

Jot down the key ideas covered in this chapter.

What has been your experience with the Holy Spirit? In what ways are you comfortable, uncomfortable, unfamiliar, or indifferent to the presence of God's Spirit in your life?

If you have children, what are some ways you may feel concern about passing down your struggle with overeating to future generations?

What are some distractions in your life that make it difficult to hear God speaking to you through the Holy Spirit? In what ways can you minimize these distractions to give the Spirit an opportunity to speak to you?

If you don't currently read and meditate on Scripture, take a moment to write a plan for committing to this in the future. At what time of day and in what place would you like to read Scripture? What passages or books of the Bible would you like to read?

_____

_____

_____

_____

In what ways would your eating habits or thoughts about your body or food (perhaps idolatry of food, health, or being thin) be considered sin and worth confessing to God?

_____

_____

_____

_____

SET FREE & SATISFIED

JOURNALING

Set a timer for five minutes and write any thoughts or reflections you have. Use the space below to write during the five minutes.

SEEK THE SPIRIT EVERY DAY

MEMORIZE

Memorize the following verse this week and write it on an index card or Post-it Note where you can see it each day. Try to say it out loud daily and commit it to memory during this week.

"If we confess our sins, (God) is faithful and just and will forgive us our sins and purify us from all unrighteousness."
—1 John 1:9

Copy this verse in the space below as you begin to commit it to memory. If you choose a different verse, write it in the space below.

_____

_____

_____

_____

_____

PRAYER

Check in with your friend who is supporting you in prayer. Take a moment to write your own prayer to God in the space on the following page. You may like to pray using language from the following passages:

- *Matthew 6:9–13 ("lead me not into temptation")*
- *1 Corinthians 10:13 ("provide a way of escape")*
- *2 Timothy 1:7 (pray for self-control)*
- *James 1:15 (ask for wisdom to use your freedom responsibly)*

PRACTICE

Remember to show yourself love and self-care. Take time today to seek the Spirit through solitude, Scripture, saying "sorry" (confession), and submitting. Use the following guide for your devotion time.

Read John 14:15–31:

- Write one verse from the passage that "speaks to you" or stands out to you.

- What does this passage tell you about what God is like?

- What does this passage tell you about what people are like?

- What is one practical way you might want to try to live differently this week because of this passage?

Finally, write a prayer to God. Ask the Lord to show you any ways you may have sinned related to your eating or your body. Write any other thoughts you'd like to share with God in your prayer. You may want to write a prayer submitting to God's good plans for your life, no matter the cost. End your prayer by writing, "Lord, please speak to me," then draw two parallel lines below this. Wait quietly and write down any words/phrases, images, or verses that come to

SEEK THE SPIRIT EVERY DAY

you below the line. Later you can refer to this and quickly know that the words below the two lines were a response to your prayer.

CHAPTER 8

Experience Life to the Full

*The thief comes only to steal and kill and destroy;
I have come that they may have life, and have it to the full.*
—John 10:10

In my weight-loss journey, I experienced periods of two extremes. At one end of the spectrum, I was obsessed with being thin, daily tracking my calories on a white board in my kitchen and starving myself with trendy diets. My friend Christine became so worried about me that she took the time to tell me. In my dysfunction, this only encouraged my efforts to know that someone had noticed how much weight I'd lost. I loved the concern and attention. As a worker at an outpatient medical office, I'd sneak into empty patient rooms multiple times a day to weigh myself. When I finally reached a size six, I accused that poor retail worker that her company had made the shorts larger. I wasn't satisfied with my new lower weight. I was thin but miserable.

That season of intense food deprivation was followed by another extreme. I'd drive to the local grocery store at night, buy an entire pack of Oreo cookies for myself, and secretly consume them with a half-gallon of milk in my parked car on a dark street. At a church retreat where people had been asked to bring homemade cookies for the opening night's social event, I roamed the large room eating so many cookies that, as I lay down to sleep that night, I felt like my brain was rattling in my skull due to the insane amount of sugar I'd consumed. Nights like these, I'd hate myself and cry as I tried to fall asleep. Another time, one of my youth ministry students noticed my bloated face the morning after a binge and asked me about it. I was overweight and miserable.

Both of these extreme lifestyles were problematic. At either end of the spectrum, I was devoted to my own destruction (Exodus 22:20). When I was super thin, I had made a god of being skinny and was in bondage to getting thin and staying thin. As I so enjoyed the admiration of others, I also see that I'd made a god of myself and the attention I could receive. I was obsessed with the size of my body, my calorie count, and whether people noticed how thin I was. In the other scenario, when I binged in secret, food was my false god that I ran to for security and comfort instead of going to God.

Jesus doesn't want us to be devoted to things that destroy us. He has a different vision for our lives. In John 10:10, He said, "The thief comes only to steal and kill and destroy; I have come that they may have life, and have it to the full." I didn't have life at all—I had thinness or I had a lot of sweets, but I didn't have life! After we have practiced waiting for (H)unger, naming our (E)motions when we want to eat but aren't hungry, and are finally pursuing intimacy with the (L)ord through the Holy Spirit, how do we successfully move from a lifestyle of destruction to a vibrant life that's full of variety, relationships, and activities that don't always center around our body and eating?

Nineteenth-century educator Charlotte Mason perfectly named the antidote to a life set on self-destruction through sinful behavior. Her approach to disciplining children was not about punishment but focused on helping children grow in their responsibility and self-control while forming good habits that would last a lifetime. That's what we want to do with our freedom with food: grow in our responsibility and form good habits. Sadly, many of us never learned to do this as kids.

Mason talked about "pursuing life" to not be devoted to things that are destructive to us. She wrote:

> If minds are interested, skills are being learned, loving relationships are enjoyed, creativity is encouraged, beauty in nature, art and music are appreciated, hours are spent in free play, and children learn to climb, swim, ride, canoe, ski or skate—why, these children will be well on the way to having their sinful natures put in the back seat! . . . Sinful natures expand like a malignancy at any age with loneliness, mental poverty, boredom, passivity, hunger, tiredness, and deprivation of daily contact with the rich source of goodness—the Word of God.[1]

Does this sound familiar? Does your overeating increase when you feel lonely, bored, or tired? You've reached the final step of Releasity: **Experience Life to the Full. This is also the "P" in**

our daily rhythm acronym, HELP: pursue life. In my life, I've experienced healing from food addiction as I've learned to eat with hunger, identify my emotions and take them to the Lord, and finally, to pursue life-giving activities that ultimately replace my desire to eat because the activities are more life-giving than the food. We can "experience life to the full" in four key areas: healing the past, having healthy relationships today, forming "happy new habits," and "hanging in for the harvest."

HEAL THE PAST

One way we experience life to the full is by healing our past. Many of us overeat because of unresolved issues that may have happened years ago. Just as you must get out of debt to develop a current healthy budget, reckoning with the wounds of your past helps you live a full life in the present and stop going to food as a way of coping.

Past pain can affect us in various ways. People may have told us lies or made hurtful comments that continue to shame us, and we eat to feel comfort. Even our current conflicts can strike a nerve because they resemble a similar past unresolved issue. I once had a boss who regularly teased and criticized me; her words sparked the insecurities I felt because of another person's words in the past. I knew the Lord was calling me to endure this relationship so He could demonstrate His presence with me, His love for me, and His desire to set me free from the fear of her or anyone like her. Do you ever have a repeated relationship challenge and suspect the Lord wants to help you overcome your fear and heal you?

We can feel negative emotions related to pain we experienced years ago. We can feel unrest now because we have insecurities or idols that began in our past. Someone may have caused us to feel rejected.

Maybe we are upset with God or feel heartache and pain because of something that happened or didn't happen. An important aspect of healing the past is acknowledging our disappointment with God. The Bible is full of accounts of people, such as Jacob and Jonah, who wrestled with God. It's important to be honest with God because He already knows what we are thinking and feeling. A "cleansing" can happen when we are honest before God about the ways we believe He has let us down. Lamenting is helpful and holy.

If we don't resolve past issues, they may negatively affect our current relationships. In some cases, we clam up and turn our sadness and anger inward. We don't speak up for ourselves and start a pattern of looking out for others' needs more than our own. Alternately, we can unleash our anger and sadness on people who do not deserve it because we are actually releasing emotions caused by someone else who hurt us in the past. If we don't deal with our pain, we may dish it out to others. As the saying goes, "Hurt people hurt people." We then have three options. We can turn the pain inward and become depressed, we can turn it outward and hurt others, or we can properly dispose of it. I suggest the third option is what God wants for us.

Jesus died on the cross to take away the pain of our past, including the pain others have caused us and the pain we have caused others. If we don't take an honest look at these events and go through a process of healing, we devalue what Jesus did on the cross. This leaves us tangled in anger and other negative emotions. We need to deal with our pain, with Jesus, to be set free from it and not become bitter. Proverbs 4:23 says, "Above all else, guard your heart, for everything you do flows from it."

God began to heal my past on a cold Thanksgiving day in 2001. Living in the DC area and away from my family in North Carolina, I had chosen to stay put for this holiday weekend. While I had plans to eat dinner with a friend's family, I spent most of the day alone, drinking coffee, reading, and taking walks along the quiet streets, a rare opportunity in this bustling city. It was divine. I remember returning from my walk and enjoying more solitude on my couch while praying. As I settled in to speak to God, an image spontaneously appeared in my mind of people carrying old furniture out of a dusty attic space. I came to understand this as a sign that God was about to take me on a journey of looking at my past to find healing and setting me free from painful emotions that still affected my present.

The process of healing my past could be summarized in one word: forgiveness. While being healed from food addiction, I came to see that I carried a lot of pain in a few relationships. My friend Lisa, a professional counselor, helped me understand that the distance between the other person and me consisted of wrongs I'd committed against them and wrongs they had committed against me. Some of these were with friends, and some were with family. While I couldn't force people to apologize to me, I could, at least, own what was mine, apologize for it, and potentially decrease some of the distance between us.

In particular, I gave time and reflection to the sins I'd committed against my father and thought about how I could ask for forgiveness when I was ready. Some of you may say, "I've been hurt by people who I really don't think I've hurt. Why would I ask them for forgiveness?" Maybe you haven't sinned against the person who hurt you, but the Bible teaches we have all sinned in some way. In Psalm 51:3-5, David wrote, "For I know my transgressions, and my sin is always before me. Against you, you only, have I sinned and done what is evil in your sight; so you are right in your verdict and justified when you judge. Surely I was sinful at birth, sinful from the time my mother conceived me."

Forgiving others and being forgiven go hand in hand. In the Lord's Prayer, Jesus instructs us to pray, "Forgive us our debts as we also have forgiven our debtors" (Matthew 6:12). Just after this, He tells us to pray that we won't be led into temptation. I can't help but wonder if there's a correlation between being forgiven, forgiving others, and subsequently being strengthened to not fall into temptation (like overeating). In Matthew 6:14–15, Jesus said, "For if you forgive other people when they sin against you, your heavenly Father will also forgive you. But if you do not forgive others their sins, your Father will not forgive your sins."

When we forgive others, we no longer hold them responsible for how they hurt us. We transfer our pain to the cross on which Jesus died for us. We don't carry the weight of the other person's wounds or bitterness. As Christians, we have a responsibility to forgive others, because God forgave our sins through Jesus's sacrifice on the cross. When you earnestly ask God to help you, He will enable you to forgive those who have hurt you, even if they never apologize.

While you may not care for the process of asking for forgiveness from others, nor about forgiving others, remember that it is beneficial to your overall well-being to "properly dispose" of your negative feelings toward a person. You don't want this pain to stay with you and cause you to accidentally pass it on to another person or cause yourself harm through self-destructive behavior. If you hold onto unforgiveness, you are the one who suffers because you will become bitter. Bitter people often become lonely people, because it's hard to keep company with a chronically unhappy person.

The forgiveness process will require intentional time for reflection. Take time to pray, process, and write about these inflictions.

Follow the prescription of Psalm 4:4: "In your anger, do not sin; when you are on your beds, search your hearts and be silent." Ask God to search your heart and show you the anxious places and offensive ways (Psalm 139:23–24) where you have been hurt and where you have hurt others. Hebrews 4:16 advises us to "approach God's throne of grace with confidence, so that we may receive mercy and find grace to help us in our time of need." God loves you, cherishes you, and accepts you as you are.

After praying for the Holy Spirit's guidance and insight and writing about the pain you have caused others and the pain you have felt, continuing to reflect on Psalm 51:6–12 is a great help. Lay your hurts, sins, and shortcomings before God as you seek Him first through this passage:

> Yet you desired faithfulness even in the womb; you
> taught me wisdom in that secret place. Cleanse me with
> hyssop, and I will be clean; wash me, and I will be whiter
> than snow. Let me hear joy and gladness; let the bones
> you have crushed rejoice. Hide your face from my sins
> and blot out all my iniquity. Create in me a pure heart,
> O God, and renew a steadfast spirit within me. Do not
> cast me from your presence or take your Holy Spirit
> from me. Restore to me the joy of your salvation and
> grant me a willing spirit, to sustain me.

Ask God for forgiveness and receive His love and grace and mercy. Remember that Jesus said there is celebrating in heaven when we repent (Luke 15:7). This is a celebration! Asking for forgiveness is good.

EXPERIENCE LIFE TO THE FULL

Next, consider if God is leading you to confess your sins directly to the person. If so, pray God will give you that opportunity and that He will work through the Holy Spirit to guide you into that conversation. God can be trusted to make this conversation happen.

Much conflict existed between my father and me when I applied to work for an international ministry organization. As part of my interview process, I participated in psychological testing, which uncovered the challenges in our relationship. My interviewers tried to explore this topic with me, but I genuinely had no idea what they were talking about. As time went on, however, I too realized there was a distance between my father and me and that we were both at fault. I had been afraid to speak honestly with him because his father, my grandfather, had committed suicide when I was young. Fearing my dad would take his own life if I opened up to him, I stayed silent for years. Even though my counselor friend encouraged me to apologize for my wrongdoings so the distance between my father and me could decrease, it still took months before I was ready and believed God was leading me to have a direct conversation with my father.

Then one day, it happened. I knew it was time to apologize. I called him with a significant time difference and an ocean between us. He happened to pick up the phone on a weekday afternoon, which was rare because he was typically working out on our farm or moving around our rural community during the day.

After the initial surprise of him answering the phone, I nervously apologized for all the offenses I could remember committing against him. I distinctly remember him saying, "Oh, don't worry about it. It's in the past." But I knew I needed to ask for forgiveness to clear my own conscience and to handle this sin in the way God prescribed. That conversation was the beginning of much healing and open communication between us. He even came to apologize for his contributions to our conflict in later years, and I'm thankful God orchestrated that reconciliation before my dad passed away ten years later.

When you have experienced God's kindness, love, and forgiveness, you are better able to show kindness toward others and forgive them. This is not to say anyone should stay in toxic, abusive relationships. Sometimes, you can own what is yours by asking for forgiveness and parting ways. Or perhaps you stay in the relationship because of the person's role in your life (such as a parent who God calls you to honor or another family member with whom you feel led to continue the relationship). However, it's wise and beneficial to be very careful about your interactions with such people and the frequency of those interactions. You can ask God to show you if you're not speaking up for yourself in these relationships because of fear or a history of unhealthy relationship dynamics.

Doing the work of forgiveness helps you live in peace. As you have difficult conversations and offer and ask for forgiveness, you can experience ever-growing freedom from that relationship's pain. I also cannot overstate the benefit of having a professional counselor help you process and navigate the wounds of past and current relationships. If you are in a position to seek these services, I encourage you to do so.

HEALTHY BONDS TODAY

As we begin to find healing from our past pains and come clean on how we have hurt others, we focus on how to have healthy relationships now. We can be honest when others hurt us and ask God to help us have wisdom about how to proceed. We can also have a friendship where others can share with us when we've hurt them. A pastor once gave my husband and me this rule for marriage: "No hitting below the belt and no wearing your belt around your neck."

We want to be kind to others and also not be so sensitive that others cannot share how we have hurt them. We want to offer a safe space where others can share their honest feedback with us.

Sometimes God will help us to "overlook an offense" (Proverbs 19:11) and privately process our pain through prayer, rather than pointing it out to the other person. However, other times, it is helpful to "wear white" as Nancy Groom describes in her book, *Heart to Heart about Men.* While she is advising women to show men the impact their sin has caused them, this can be a helpful tool in some of our relationships where we have experienced hurt. Groom writes, "We do not do (men) honor by ignoring their unkind or ungodly behavior. . . . We give evidence of our respect for men not by bringing them the consequences of their sin, but by showing them the consequences of their sin as it affects us. . . . In short, we can bleed when they wound our hearts—not to make them pay for their sin but to let them see what their sin has done."[2] Similar to this "wearing white," sometimes God may guide us to simply let someone know when they have hurt us.

Thankfully, we can say a simple sentence to let someone know a wrong was committed. For example, "When you (*action that was harmful*), I felt (*emotion you felt*)." This script isn't always easy to deliver, but it is helpful for formulating your thoughts and letting the person know how they affected you. Unless the person lies and denies doing what you said (and some will try!), they can't easily tell you that you don't feel what you feel. Simply naming how someone else's words or actions made you feel helps you direct the truth of the pain to someone outside of you, rather than denying it by overeating or even by acknowledging it and overeating. Having these difficult conversations is best accompanied by an internal prayer of "Come, Holy Spirit" while we interact with the person.

A red flag may develop in these types of conversations. If you find yourself in a relationship where you are constantly accused of causing offense when compared with your behavior in other relationships, you may be in a situation with a friend whose sensitivity may be elevated. Consider if moving forward in friendship is healthy for the two of you. In these rare cases, it may be best to own your offenses and part ways to avoid further strife for you and the other person.

Pursuing healthy present relationships is key when it comes to overcoming your struggle with food. According to one source, a common trait of people who maintain long-term weight loss is the presence of healthy attachment in relationships.[3] Anecdotally, I have witnessed this in Releasity as well. The women who come through the program with close relationships have had more success maintaining healthy eating habits than women who live alone or tend to isolate themselves. As you examine the health of your current relationships, here are some questions to ask:

- Do you have **real, in-person friendships,** or has your relationship pool been reduced to social media connections? Consider if social media has negatively affected your in-person relationships. In *Loving Your Friend Through Cancer,* Marissa Henley writes, "In our social-media-obsessed culture, we often have a skewed perspective of the closeness of our friendships. Just because you know what your friend ate for dinner last night doesn't mean you are in her small circle of best friends. . . . Inner-circle friends talk, text, or visit frequently. Deeper discussions about your family, emotions, joys, and struggles form an essential aspect of your friendship. You know each other's loved ones well.

You are familiar with each other's likes, dislikes, favorites, preferences and personalities."[4]

- Are your **friendships healthy**? Or do you have some key relationships that would be considered "codependent"? These are relationships where you might feel afraid of someone or feel that they are controlling you. Perhaps you don't fully trust the other person, or you don't feel like you can speak up for what you need in the relationship. On the flip side, you may be the person who is controlling, and another person lives in fear of you. The Bible says, "Perfect love drives out fear" (1 John 4:18), and relationships that have fear as an element are not healthy ones. A popular book on this topic, *Codependent No More,* by Melody Beattie, may be beneficial to read if you find yourself in this kind of relationship. *Boundaries*, by Dr. Henry Cloud and Dr. John Townsend, also delves into how to form healthy relationships.

- Are you in friendships where you can be your **authentic self?** Because of what Jesus did for us on the cross, making us perfect and righteous in the sight of a Holy God, we don't have to pretend to be perfect for people. We can be vulnerable with trusted friends. It is when we go below the surface and share our honest thoughts and feelings with others that we build true intimacy in our friendships.

- Are you taking the **initiative to make friends** by going to groups where you can meet people with similar interests? Can you check out church small groups, or invite people over for simple visits? Often, addictive behavior such as overeating can lead us to isolate ourselves, which only makes our pull to the refrigerator stronger. If you live alone, consider making a habit of reaching out to meet up with someone or participate in a social activity at least once a week to ensure you are spending time in social situations. While pets are cute and fun to snuggle with, it's important to have quality human friendships. Search for local meet-ups with people who share your interests, find opportunities to volunteer where you will meet people, and ask God to guide you to fulfilling friendships.

HAPPY NEW HABITS

We have already talked about the importance of finding alternative activities for when we want to eat but don't feel physically hungry. In Chapter Five, you began keeping a list of new, healthy alternatives for eating when you craved food but weren't physically hungry. This list will help you as you begin to pursue the full life Jesus wants for you, one where you aren't stuck in the kitchen overeating, then stuck in your bed feeling guilty about what you overate.

In the back of this book, you'll find a "Happy New Habits" checklist with ideas for how to spend your time when you want to eat but don't feel physically hungry. You can also download one in color through the Releasity website. These activities cover the following nine categories:

- practicing self-care
- being creative
- learning
- spending time in nature
- enjoying movement

EXPERIENCE LIFE TO THE FULL

- building relationships
- growing in faith
- playing
- serving others

Posting and memorizing these categories for activities will help you shift to them in times of temptation. I encourage you to spend a fun and relaxing day or evening inviting friends over to pursue these activities together. You'll also want to keep a list of additional diversions that uniquely appeal to you. A few of the habits are worth a quick discussion.

Self-care is a powerful alternative to overeating. Sadly, many of us have neglected self-care because we do not like our bodies or we feel impatient when performing the tasks. When we take the time to do nice things for our bodies, we are showing gratitude for how our bodies are "fearfully and wonderfully made" (Psalm 139:14). Kathleen Norris wrote in *Quotidian Mysteries*,

> The comfortable lies we tell ourselves regarding these "little things"—that they don't matter, and that daily personal and household chores are of no significance to us spiritually—are exposed as falsehoods when we consider that reluctance to care for the body is one of the first symptoms of extreme melancholia. Shampooing the hair, washing the body, brushing the teeth, drinking enough water, taking a daily vitamin, going for a walk, as simple as they seem, are acts of self-respect. They enhance one's ability to take pleasure in oneself and in the world.[5]

To make this time for ourselves, we must find ways to say "no" to competing activities. I once heard a man commend his wife because she "never says 'no' to anyone." My first thought was, "Oh, dear! That's not good!" Sometimes we must say "no" to requests and invitations, so we can say "yes" to our own health and personal goals.

Sensory delights can also help us move past overeating. Since eating is a sensory experience, other such experiences may provide helpful diversions when we want to eat but aren't hungry. Light a candle to enjoy the smell, sit by a fire and feel the heat, snuggle under a cozy blanket as it warms your skin, take a hot bath, listen to calming music, or spend time in nature while enjoying the sounds of singing birds and feeling the warmth of the sun or the breeze. Often, if we take the time to explore other sensory pleasures, the appeal of overeating will fade. The lie that food will fix our problems is further exposed when we take delight in God's creation through means that don't add calories and weight to our bodies.

The diversion of serving others comes with a biblical promise. Proverbs 11:25 says, "A generous person will prosper; whoever refreshes others will be refreshed." My sister bravely battled cancer when she was a young mom. While caring for her children during one of her medical appointments, I heard a knock on her door. As I looked out the window, I noticed her neighbor holding a small container of soup. Accustomed to people delivering family-sized meals for my sister's family of four, I admit I was a bit thrown off and thought, *That's nice of this woman, but does she really think this small cup of soup will feed the whole family?* I politely thanked the neighbor and carried the soup to the refrigerator. Years later, I learned the whole story. The neighbor had lost her son in a tragic accident during his first semester of college. On the anniversary of his death, she makes a point to do something for someone else to take her mind off her grief, if only for a short time. Her small cup of soup offered a meal for my sister and a lifelong lesson for me.

HANG IN FOR THE HARVEST

We are now in the final phase of following the Releasity approach to eating. As Winston Churchill said, "Now this is not the end. It is not even the beginning of the end. But it is, perhaps, the end of the beginning." As we explore the last aspect of Experiencing Life to the Full, let's talk about how to "Hang in for the Harvest" and persevere in this new approach to food, no matter the obstacles and challenges we face going forward. As Galatians 6:9 says, "Let us not become weary in doing good, for at the proper time we will reap a harvest if we do not give up." Let's enjoy that harvest!

At this point, you might be sensing with your freedom that it would be good to have a specific plan for how to proceed from here, and I agree. Plans can be useful for having "tools, not rules" and provide a nice guardrail when we are setting new goals. At Christmastime, I'm reminded that even God had a plan in sending Jesus to save the world from our sins. Throughout the Old Testament, we see the plan unfolding as multiple prophets point to the coming Messiah. Plans are good, and making a plan for how to move forward with your food freedom is essential.

Remember the process will take time, but we will know the resulting change is thorough and authentic because it stands the test of time. We will also learn so much in the process that we can later pass on to help others. I believe God wants to develop wonderful character traits in us, including perseverance, patience, hope, and trust. When we persevere in the process of healing, we grow in our character. We also grow closer to God as we struggle and learn to lean on Him for support and direction.

If you are discouraged when considering that this process will take longer than you want it to, think about a situation where it is better for someone to take their time and do something slowly rather than quickly. Women in the Releasity course have named painting your nails, baking something from scratch, choosing a car, and writing a will. Likewise, an educator talked about the importance of taking your time when taking a test, quoting a popular refrain in her classroom: "The first in the tray doesn't always get an A!"

Releasity's logo is a butterfly. Admittedly, I chose it because butterflies are beautiful and represent freedom in their ability to break out of the cocoon and fly away. Recently, as I took a deeper look, I realized the transformation of a caterpillar to a butterfly is a complex process with even more similarities to our being liberated from overeating than I first recognized. Moreover, the caterpillar's journey to freedom has been described as complicated, gruesome, and fascinating, words I'd use to explain my own healing transformation.

It's almost laughable how much a caterpillar's change resembles our experience with food. First, caterpillars eat a ton of food before they even begin their transformation in the chrysalis. I don't know about you, but I had that step easily covered before my transformation! Second, when caterpillars begin their metamorphosis, they go into isolation. Does this remind you of those moments of sneaking food when you are alone, then feeling terrible afterward? The butterfly's transformation involves shedding multiple outer layers and turning "soupy" on the inside as they become a new creation. Shedding these layers is similar to getting at the root causes of our overeating so we can find healing. Those tears we cry can even feel a little "soupy" sometimes, can't they?

The transformation period from caterpillar to butterfly is not a short blip in their overall lifespans. Let's have some fun with the math. For example, the red admiral butterfly's average total life span is fifty-six days, and its time in the chrysalis stage (the isolated, soupy, shedding-layers phase) is ten days. That means it spends roughly 20 percent of its whole life being transformed. In human years, with the average life expectancy being seventy-three years (as of 2019),[6] that would translate to about fourteen years. A monarch butterfly is a little more fortunate. Its total life span is roughly 210 days with the transformation phase lasting twelve days. That accounts for 6 percent of its entire life and, translated to the average human life expectancy, would equal about four years.

I know we can't fully compare our change to butterflies, but the numbers aren't that far off in terms of percentage of your total life span. Women often ask me how long my process took, because they want to know what to expect for themselves. Unfortunately, I can't successfully predict that. But I will say the transformation and healing process lasted seven years for me, from the fall of 2000 until 2007. Interestingly, the number seven is symbolic in near Eastern and Israelite literature, including the Scriptures of the Bible. The number communicates a sense of fullness, completeness, or perfection.

I once owned a printer that had the option of printing documents in "fast draft" mode or "normal" mode. If I didn't care about the quality of the job because it was a draft or it wasn't something to be shared with other people, I quickly chose "fast draft" to save ink. I used the "normal" mode for the important print jobs. Similarly, in the process of being set free from overeating, it's important to take the "normal" and complete version. I hope you'll continue this journey with a desire to experience your transformation well, in a way that is authentic, thorough, and lasting. If this were a piece of meat, trust me, you'd want the well-done version!

For this reason, Paul prayed for the church at Colossae to have endurance and patience as they grew in their faith. He wanted them to have a strong, complete, and mature relationship with God and existence as a church body. Colossians 1:9–12 says:

> We continually ask God to fill you with the knowledge
> of his will through all the wisdom and understanding
> that the Spirit gives, so that you may live a life worthy
> of the Lord and please him in every way: bearing fruit
> in every good work, growing in the knowledge of God,
> being strengthened with all power according to his
> glorious might so that you may have great endurance
> and patience, and giving joyful thanks to the Father, who
> has qualified you to share in the inheritance of his holy
> people in the kingdom of light.

The Centers for Disease Control (CDC) concurs with the importance of taking your time to achieve lasting change with your health. A CDC report states that people who lose weight gradually and steadily (about one to two pounds per week) are more successful at keeping weight off long-term.[7] How can we do this? That same CDC report references the National Weight Control Registry,[8] which collects data on people who have lost five percent to ten percent of their body weight and kept it off for five to ten years. Let's return to the number seven as I share seven common characteristics of successful participants noted in these studies.[9]

PHYSICALLY ACTIVE LIFESTYLE

Don't worry! You don't have to be a super athlete to have an active lifestyle! Research shows that walking is the most common trait among people who maintain long-term weight loss. Remember that you can just throw on your socks and sneakers to take a walk; no fancy exercise equipment or gear is needed. I find it helpful to think in terms of "minutes out" and "minutes back." Ten minutes out on a walk, then ten minutes back can fit in to most busy lifestyles if it's a priority. Even the smallest movement, something that is "incompatible with eating," will help steer you away from excess food. A counselor once encouraged me to find something small that I could enjoy with my fingers as a starting place for activity. Perhaps you'd enjoy painting, playing an instrument, or writing.

INTENTIONALITY AND TRACKING

I've only reached my ideal weight range twice in my life without effort. Once, I was clinically depressed, and the other time I was falling in love with my husband. I don't want to repeat clinical depression and I can't replicate the experience of meeting and falling in love with my husband for the first time. We must be intentional with our health. Now that you've learned the steps of Releasity, you'll probably want to make a plan for the kinds of foods you'd like to eat, the times you'll take a walk, or how you'll seek accountability from a friend. Keeping track of something in this process can help you stay focused. This "keeping track" doesn't need to involve your weight if that makes you uncomfortable. You can track the number of times you walk in a week, how many glasses of water you drink, or how often you wait for hunger before eating in a day. Tracking something helps you remember that you care about this struggle. It also helps you pay attention to your choices throughout the day. Remember, this practice of tracking is a "tool, not a rule."

GRATITUDE

People who are grateful for the victories, both small and large, are more likely to have long-term success with weight management. I love to hear women at Releasity share their gratitude that they are continuing to participate in the group, that they are perservering, and that God hasn't given up on them. We can be grateful for so many blessings at any size. You may want to keep a gratitude journal and write at least three things you're thankful for each night. The data confirms that gratitude has documented benefits.

INTERNAL LOCUS OF CONTROL

People who believe they have the power to change within them (and that it doesn't lie in some external program, person, or diet) also tend to have long-term success. This is commonly referred to as "agency." In the Releasity approach, we believe the power of God's Spirit is working in us to bring this lasting change.

OPTIMISM AND POSITIVE RELATIONSHIPS

National Weight Control Registry members have a hopeful outlook and are securely attached in healthy relationships. They are generally not depressed, which is why it's important to seek counseling and/ or medical attention if you feel that you are struggling with depression. Having a friend to call is crucial for conversation, shared prayer, walks, or a meal together. The companionship of friends helped carry me through my darkest days, especially while I was being healed of disordered binge eating.

LOW NOVELTY SEEKING

Those who experience long-term success are ones who are not always seeking something new to experience. For those of us who do struggle with overeating, this may be an indicator that we are novelty seeking. We must make the most of our "happy new habits" to have outlets for new experiences rather than going to food for thrills and entertainment.

AWARENESS OF BENEFITS

Remember how we started this process by naming what we wanted and why we wanted it? It's helpful to keep in mind the benefits that will come as you wait for hunger and seek God to comfort you and guide you when you want to eat without hunger. Keeping a list of why you want this change is critical.

As we wrap up this stage of learning a new way to approach food, let me remind you that you *can* do what has been covered in this book. You have already read this book to the end, inviting God into your struggle with food and letting the contents of the chapters settle into your thoughts as you go about your day. Furthermore, God promises to help you. 1 Thessalonians 5:24 says, "The one who calls you is faithful, and he will do it." In Exodus 14:14, we read His promise, "The Lord will fight for you; you need only to be still."

Remember to keep revisiting and practicing the steps of Releasity:

- **Remember** What You Want.

- **Expect** the Lord to Heal.

- **Live** Out of Your Freedom.

- **Eat** with Hunger When You Feel It.

- **Acknowledge** Your Emotions.

- **Seek** the Spirit Every Day.

- **Experience** Life to the Full.

This is the **Releasity** way!

God will keep moving you forward on this healing journey if you keep seeking Him. The other good news is that it won't always be this hard. Similar to learning how to drive a car with a stick shift, the steps that take so much intentionality now will become second nature with enough time and transformation. Stay in step with the Spirit, stay in community with friends who can support you, and you will reap the harvest if you don't give up. Be curious, not critical. Remember that kinder is faster. Most of all, don't forget that this way of life is not self-help—it's Holy Spirit help. The power that raised Jesus Christ from the dead is the same power at work in you today!

A PRAYER FOR YOU

As we conclude, this is my prayer for you, which comes from Ephesians 1:15–22:

> For this reason, ever since I heard about your faith in the Lord Jesus and your love for all the saints, I have not stopped giving thanks for you, remembering you

in my prayers. I keep asking that the God of our Lord Jesus Christ, the glorious Father, may give you the Spirit of wisdom and revelation, so that you may know him better. I pray that the eyes of your heart may be enlightened in order that you may know the hope to which he has called you, the riches of His glorious inheritance in his holy people, and his incomparably great power for us who believe. That power is the same as the mighty strength he exerted when he raised Christ from the dead and seated him at his right hand in the heavenly realm, far above all rule and authority, power and dominion, and every name that is invoked, not only in the present age but also in the one to come.

Amen! May it be so!

SET FREE & SATISFIED

REFLECTION QUESTIONS

Jot down the key ideas covered in this chapter.

_____

_____

_____

_____

When you think of "healing the past" as it relates to your eating habits, what are some examples of past offenses or wounds that may have led you to overeat?

_____

_____

_____

_____

As you read about "healing the past," did any specific relationships or offenses come to mind? If so, in what circumstances or among which people might you consider asking for forgiveness or offering forgiveness for past wounds?

_____

_____

_____

_____

Reflect on the state of your current relationships. Who are some trusted friends with whom you enjoy quality time and can share your honest thoughts and be yourself? How has the rise of online "friendships" impacted the closeness of your in-person friendships? If this is an area where you'd benefit from developing true friendships, what are

EXPERIENCE LIFE TO THE FULL

some specific ways you can meet like-minded friends?

_____

_____

_____

_____

Considering the list of seven common characteristics
of people who are successful with weight management,
which of these do you find most obtainable or, con-
versely, most challenging? Take a moment to ask God for
help in this area.

_____

_____

_____

_____

JOURNALING

Set a timer for five minutes and write any thoughts or reflections you
have after reading this chapter. Include any new insight gained from
this book or apart from this book. You may want to write down any
recent challenges or victories you have experienced related to your
body, eating, or your emotions. Use the space below to write during
the five minutes.

_____

_____

_____

_____

_____

_____

_____

_____

_____

_____

_____

_____

_____

_____

_____

_____

_____

_____

_____

_____

_____

_____

_____

_____

_____

MEMORIZE

Memorize one of the following verses (or a verse of your choice) and write it on an index card or Post-it Note where you can see it each day. Try to say it out loud daily and commit it to memory this week.

"The thief comes only to steal and kill and destroy; I have come that they may have life, and have it to the full."
—John 10:10

"Let us not become weary in doing good, for at the proper time we will reap a harvest if we do not give up."
—Galatians 6:9

Copy this verse in the space below as you begin to commit it to memory. If you choose a different verse, write it in the space below.

PRAYER

Check in with your friend who is supporting you in prayer. Take a moment to write your own prayer to God in the space below, giving special consideration to healing your past, having healthy relationships today, developing new habits to replace overeating, and "hanging in for the harvest."

PRACTICE

Remember to show yourself love and self-care. Post the "Happy New Habits" checklist and try at least one activity this week. As you discover diversions that will take your mind off overeating, add your own ideas, or look into classes in areas that interest you.

Next Steps

Congratulations! You've finished the first stage of exploring a new way of approaching food through the Releasity program. Don't stop here, though. Many other wonderful next steps can help you be successful on your journey. Some of these steps might be:

Continue meeting together. Hebrews 10:25 tells us the importance of continuing to come together with like-minded people for encouragement. If you have met to discuss Releasity with a formal group, your group may enjoy getting together to review key concepts, share with each other, and to pray for each other. If you've met informally with a friend or two to discuss Releasity, you may also enjoy continuing to meet to review concepts and explore freedom from food on a deeper level.

Seek professional help. Throughout this book, you've read about counselors, nutritionists, dietitians, and the like. I highly recommend tailoring your journey by meeting with these types of professionals to explore your unique circumstances and needs. Also, check with your employer's Human Resources department to learn if your health insurance program offers complimentary services of health and wellness coaches, dietitians, or discounted counseling services. Many untapped resources may be waiting for you even now.

Keep reading. Throughout my healing, I continued to discover various authors and books that helped teach me the concepts highlighted in this book. You can find books about intuitive eating, mindful eating, and emotional eating that will offer further insight. Books linking faith and addiction, as well as books about enslaving idols, are also related to this topic. Visit **www.joymast.com** for current recommendations of book titles and authors.

Write regularly. While reading this book, you practiced pausing for five minutes to write down your thoughts. Don't stop! Writing our thoughts and feelings can be highly therapeutic. Set a timer for five minutes on a daily basis, and grab a pen and paper to help calm your mind and bring order to your thoughts as you also release them to God.

Seek the Spirit. Our hearts were designed to love God and love people. Make sure to dedicate regular time to seeking God through prayer, reading Scripture, worshipping, memorizing and meditating on Bible verses, and having fellowship with other Christians.

Make a plan. As you begin to enjoy your freedom with food, you will likely join many other women who have realized they actually don't like how they feel after eating too much. With your freedom, develop a plan for how you'd like to pursue health moving forward. Remember that your plan is a system for success, not another round of restricting yourself in a way that will cause you to rebound. This plan, or system, is a set of "tools, not rules!" Women who have completed the Releasity course have found it beneficial to continue meeting weekly to make a practical plan for the upcoming week. Using the acronym "GEM," which stands for "God, Eat, and Move," they share insight from the previous week, then take time to talk about how and when they will spend time with God during the upcoming week. They also make a practical plan for how they want to eat and specify when and how will they make time for exercise they enjoy. Sharing ideas out loud and asking for accountability helps women gain traction in this new way of living.

ADDITIONAL RESOURCES

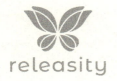

EMOTIONS WHEEL

I want to eat but I'm not hungry.
What am I feeling?

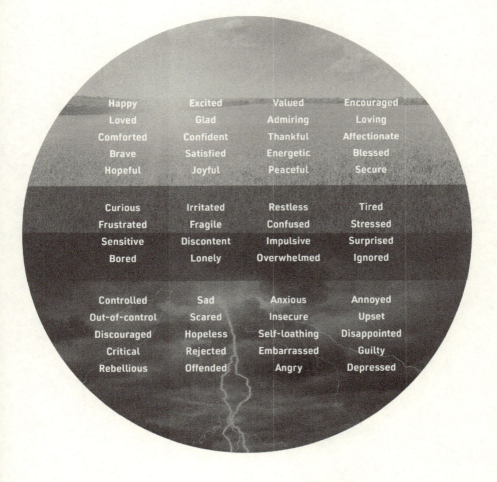

WWW.RELEASITY.ORG

ADDITIONAL RESOURCES

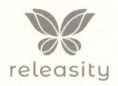

PURSUE LIFE

Happy New Habits

"I have come that they may have life and have it to the full." —JOHN 10:10

Self-Care

Moisturize your heels, schedule a medical check-up, or drink a glass of water.

Create

Play an instrument, build something, organize, paint or knit.

Learning

Study something new, visit a museum or read a non-fiction book.

Nature

Take a walk, sit outside, tend to plants, and enjoy the outdoors.

Movement

Exercise in a way that you enjoy. Keep it up for at least 10 minutes.

Relationships

Go beyond texting and social media by visiting or calling a friend.

Faith

Spend time alone with God, read your Bible, write your thoughts and prayers.

Play

Have fun and relax! Read a book or magazine, take a bath, watch a movie.

Service

Do something to serve someone else in your home or community.

WWW.RELEASITY.ORG

SET FREE & SATISFIED

BIBLE STUDY PASSAGES: WHO GOD IS

Read the following Bible verses that describe God's character. Using an online thesaurus, write an antonym (a word of opposite meaning) for each character trait of God. Honestly consider if your view of God agrees with what the Bible says or if you have a misperception of God.

God's Character Traits	Antonym
Gracious, compassionate, slow to anger, rich in love, kind (Psalm 145:8, John 17:23, Lamentations 3:22, Psalm 103:8–13)	*Example: Unkind, angry*
Near to me and listening (Psalm 34:18, Psalm 66:17-20)	
Counselor, teacher (John 14:26-27)	
Pleased and delighting in me (Zephaniah 3:17, Ephesians 1:5)	
Present, always with me, wants to be with me (Deuteronomy 31:6, John 17:24)	
Patient (2 Peter 3:9)	

ADDITIONAL RESOURCES

Tender, gentle (Isaiah 42:1–3)	
Trustworthy (2 Timothy 1:12)	
Satisfies our desires (Psalm 81:10, Psalm 34:8)	
Sovereign (Job 42:1–2)	
Has good plans for me (Jeremiah 29:11, John 14:1–3)	
Forgiving (1 John 1:9)	
Understands my weakness (Psalm 103:14)	

SET FREE & SATISFIED

BIBLE STUDY PASSAGES:
WHO I AM

Read the following Bible verses that describe who you are because of
Christ. Honestly consider if your view of yourself agrees with what
the Bible says or if you have an inaccurate view of yourself.

Who I Am Because of Christ	My Self-Perception
New creation (2 Corinthians 5:17)	
Loved (Romans 8:38–39)	
Free from condemnation (Romans 8:1–2)	
Forgiven (Colossians 3:13)	
Purified (1 John 1:9)	
Without shame (Isaiah 54:4–5, Psalm 34:4–5)	
Child of God (John 1:12)	
Delighted in (Zephaniah 3:17)	

ADDITIONAL RESOURCES

Jesus's friend (John 15:14)	
In fellowship with Jesus (Revelation 3:20)	
Released from captivity (Isaiah 61:1)	
Justified by faith (Romans 5:1–2)	
Having God's peace (Isaiah 26:3, John 14:27)	
Comforted (2 Corinthians 1:3–4)	

ACKNOWLEDGMENTS

To Threasa Lambert, who first believed in me and helped me start the Releasity course. Thank you for your support as I welcomed the first groups of women to explore these concepts.

To Julie Foldesi, my creativity accountability partner and COVID Quarantine Buddy ("QB"), who stayed by my side for each stage of bringing this book to the finish line.

To Kathy Izard, Niki Hardy, and Rob Baddorf, for coaching me and helping me turn my thoughts into action and removing my barriers.

To the women who have already taken the Releasity course in person and who kept telling me I needed to write the book—this is for you.

To the readers of this book's manuscript who gave me honest, constructive feedback: Danielle, Katie, April, Libba, Heather, Michele, Rebecca, Joy, and Anne. Thank you for your sacrifice of time and the gift of your minds to make this a better experience for all readers.

To the women who have faithfully prayed for the course, its participants, and my leadership over the past decade, your petitions to heaven have torn down strongholds.

To Kathy Brown, for your honesty and faithfulness in editing this book, a dream come true that I can hold in my hands forever.

Thank you to Patrice Gopo and Joy Callaway, fellow authors who offered wise and generous counsel.

Finally, to my family: Steve, thank you for giving so many hours to designing the website, the printable materials, course workbook, and this book. Your gift with design, photography, videos, and art have taken Releasity to the next level. And to Greta and Elizabeth, thank you for supporting and welcoming Releasity as the fifth member of our family. May this book inspire you to pursue your own dreams in life!

NOTES

Introduction

1 James Clear, *Atomic Habits: An Easy & Proven Way to Build Good Habits & Break Bad Ones* (New York: Avery, 2018).

Chapter One

1 "Medical Weight Management | Nutrition and Weight Management," Boston Medical Center, accessed January 18, 2023, https://www.bmc.org/nutrition-and-weight-management.

2 "Why People Diet, Lose Weight and Gain It All Back," Cleveland Clinic Health Essentials, 2019, https://health.clevelandclinic.org/why-people-diet-lose-weight-and-gain-it-all-back/.

Chapter Two

1 "Current Cigarette Smoking Among Adults in the United States," CDC, https://www.cdc.gov/tobacco/data_statistics/fact_sheets/adult_data/cig_smoking/index.htm.

Chapter Three

1 "Lent Day 24: The Branch," Gospel in Life, accessed January 22, 2023, https://gospelinlife.com/lent-devotional/lent-day-24-the-branch/.

2 Lou Priolo, *The Heart of Anger: Practical Help for the Prevention and Cure of Anger in Children* (Conway, AR: Grace & Truth Books, 2015), p. 43.

Chapter Four

1 "Fast Food Restaurants," The American Customer Satisfaction Index, accessed April 7, 2023, http://www.theacsi.org/industries/restaurant/fast-food/.

2 Elyse Resch and Evelyn Tribole, *Intuitive Eating, 4th Edition: A Revolutionary Anti-Diet Approach* (New York: St. Martin's Publishing Group, 2020).

3 Ghislaine Schyns et al, "Exposure Therapy vs Lifestyle Intervention to Reduce Food Cue Reactivity and Binge Eating in Obesity: A Pilot Study," *Journal of Behavior Therapy and Experimental Psychology,* issue 67, June 2020, https://doi.org/10.1016/j.jbtep.2019.01.005.

Chapter Five

1 Resch and Tribole, *Intuitive Eating.*

2 "Food Tastes Stronger When You're Hungry," *ScienceDaily*, 2004, https://www.sciencedaily.com/releases/2004/02/040223072835.htm.

Chapter Six

1 *Shadowlands*, featuring Anthony Hopkins (Los Angeles, CA: Price Entertainment, 1993).

2 Sarah Haurin, "Understanding the Link Between ADHD and Binge Eating Could Point to New Treatments," Duke Research Blog, 2018, https://researchblog.duke.edu/2018/03/13/binge-eating-disorder/.

3 "Brain Reward Response Linked to Binge Eating and ADHD," CHADD, accessed January 21, 2023, https://chadd.org/adhd-news/adhd-news-adults/brain-reward-response-linked-to-binge-eating-and-adhd/.

4 Gerald G. May, *Addiction and Grace: Love and Spirituality in the Healing of Addictions* (New York: HarperCollins, 2007).

Chapter Seven

1 Joshua Choonmin Kang, *Scripture By Heart: Devotional Practicies for Memorizing God's Word* (Downers Grove, IL: InterVarsity Press, 2010).

2 Dietrich Bonhoeffer, *Life Together: The Classic Exploration of Christian Community*, trans. John W. Doberstein (New York: HarperCollins, 1954).

Chapter Eight

1 Susan S. Macaulay, *For the Children's Sake: Foundations of Education for Home and School* (Wheaton, IL: Crossway Books, 1984).

2 Nancy Groom, *Heart to Heart about Men: Words of Encouragement for Women of Integrity* (Colorado Springs, CO: NavPress, 1995).

3 Luca Montesi et al, "Long-term Weight Loss Maintenance for Obesity: A Multidisciplinary Approach," *Diabetes, Metabolic Syndrome and Obesity* vol. 2016:9 (February 2016): 37–46, https://doi.org/10.2147/DMSO.S89836.

4 Marissa L. Henley, *Loving Your Friend Through Cancer: Words and Action That Communicate Compassion* (Createspace Independent Publishing, 2016).

5 Kathleen Norris, *The Quotidian Mysteries: Laundry, Liturgy, and "Women's Work"* (Mahwah, NJ: Paulist Press, 1998).

6 "Life Tables," World Health Organization (WHO), accessed March 26, 2023, https://www.who.int/data/gho/data/themes/mortality-and-global-health-estimates/ghe-life-expectancy-and-healthy-life-expectancy.

7 "Losing Weight," Centers for Disease Control, last modified September 2022, https://www.cdc.gov/healthyweight/losing_weight/index.html.

8 National Weight Control Registry: http://www.nwcr.ws.

9 Rena R. Wing and Suzanne Phelan, "Long-term Weight Loss Maintenance," *The American Journal of Clinical Nutrition* vol. 82, no. 1 (July 2005): 222S-225, https://doi.org/10.1093/ajcn/82.1.222S.

Made in the USA
Las Vegas, NV
19 November 2023